Charles ONANA

Health legislation and hospital management

Charles ONANA

Health legislation and hospital management

A case study conducted at the Yaoundé University Hospital.

ScienciaScripts

Imprint
Any brand names and product names mentioned in this book are subject to trademark, brand or patent protection and are trademarks or registered trademarks of their respective holders. The use of brand names, product names, common names, trade names, product descriptions etc. even without a particular marking in this work is in no way to be construed to mean that such names may be regarded as unrestricted in respect of trademark and brand protection legislation and could thus be used by anyone.

Cover image: www.ingimage.com

This book is a translation from the original published under ISBN 978-620-3-45577-9.

Publisher:
Sciencia Scripts
is a trademark of
Dodo Books Indian Ocean Ltd. and OmniScriptum S.R.L publishing group

120 High Road, East Finchley, London, N2 9ED, United Kingdom
Str. Armeneasca 28/1, office 1, Chisinau MD-2012, Republic of Moldova, Europe
Printed at: see last page
ISBN: 978-620-5-93710-5

AUTHOR'S NOTE

This book is the result of research work in Hospital and Health Management that led to a Master's degree at the Catholic University of Central Africa. Initially focused on the Impact of health legislation in the management of the CHU, the theme of this work was revised after the defense and the author preferred for publication a more concise theme: Health legislation and hospital management. A case study conducted at the University Hospital in 2015. The research authorizations had been signed for the realization of this fieldwork. The years have passed, the managerial staff has changed and, perhaps, the practices too. This book does not reflect the current state of the management of the University Hospital but, on the contrary, the impact that health legislation would have in hospital management.Health legislation would then have an impact on the management of a health facility, regardless of its nature, size and missions. This impact can be positive or negative depending on whether the legislation is well or poorly applied. Within the framework of our study, our main objective was to analyze the impact of health legislation on the management of the Yaoundé University Hospital Center (CHUY) in order to improve practices related to the mastery and application of existing standards, to improve the management of the center and to boost its growth. This was a qualitative study during which 12 staff members responded to our interview on the different themes or articulations of our work. The data were collected using a semi-directive interview guide and a non-participant observation grid. They showed that there is a large number of legal texts applicable to first category hospitals. These texts are intended to organize and regulate the hospital sub-sector. However, the application of these texts by non-competent human resources is controversial at the CHUY and produces negative effects in the management of the center. All this compromises the achievement of the results of the center. The CHUY would then benefit from respecting the norms and involving all the personnel in its management without distinction or discrimination based on gender, ethnicity, religion and even political preferences. It is therefore necessary for CHUY to use **its** best human resources so that the legislation can be applied and boost its managerial efficiency.

INTRODUCTION

Hospital management is still a major concern for developing countries. These countries, which for a long time remained faithful to the old management techniques left by the colonists[1]Most of these countries are beginning to take an interest in modern management practices imposed by the modernization of the production and management systems of States. In this perspective, Cameroon has been engaged for several years in a drive to train executives and managers of hospital and health structures through public and private institutions and specialized programs. The training programs for **hospital administrators** at the National School of Administration and Magistracy (ENAM) and for **hospital and health managers at the** School of Health Sciences of the Catholic University of Central Africa (ESS/UCAC) are part of this logic.Thus, we propose to make our modest contribution to improving the management of our health facilities. It is important to remember that our hospitals still apply on a daily basis, to agree with Ateba Eyene (2010), a "management of opacity[2]"This type of management is decried by the World Health Organization (WHO). This type of management decried by the aforementioned author is most often out of phase with the legislation in force in African countries and particularly in Cameroon. Our research, as previously noted, has focused on "the impact of health legislation on the management of the Yaoundé University Hospital Center". This theme has two motives: health legislation and the management of the CHUY which is a first class hospital in Cameroon. The first motive, health legislation is the field of laws and regulations intended to standardize a sector or a field of activity. The second is an activity that consists of increasing the productivity, effectiveness and efficiency of an organization. The existing relationship between the two is proven when we know that in order to reach a high level of development, sound managerial practices are needed, which can be the result of a legal planning established beforehand or arranged on a daily basis. Thus, legislation and management become They are inseparable in that legislation shapes management and management uses legislation to establish, confirm and develop itself. In light of the above, this study attempts to understand the interactions that exist between health legislation and the management of a first class health facility such as CHUY. It aims in a qualitative **"case study"** approach to analyze the impact of health legislation in the management of CHUY. The major difficulty lay in the choice of informants and their ability to provide clear and honest information. Our work is organized into five chapters. The first chapter deals with the framework of the study, the problem and the problematic, and provides a general scientific overview of the study. The second chapter is devoted to the theoretical and conceptual framework of the study while the third chapter highlights the methodological approach of the study. The fourth chapter presents and analyzes the results. The fifth and final chapter summarizes and discusses the results.

CHAPTER 1
FRAMEWORK OF THE STUDY, PROBLEM AND ISSUES

1.1. Rationale for the choice of the study topic

According to Dépelteau (2000), five factors can guide the choice of topic. These are the researcher's personal experience and tastes, his or her strategic interests, the usefulness of the subject concerned, the development of science and the summary results of an exploratory research. These factors can justify the researcher's personal choice on the one hand and the scientific reasons on the other.

1.1.1. Personal justification

Nkoum (2005) writes about the birth of a theme that a problem generally arises from a dissatisfaction, a lack, a doubt, a difficulty, a frequency or an original idea. It is in this order of idea that the birth of the theme which relates to the incidence of the sanitary legislation in the management of the Hospital and University Center of Yaoundé is registered. Indeed, the dissatisfaction in the management of health and hospital services (strikes, bad governance, poor leadership) gave rise to the concern to study the contours and impact that legal texts can have in the health sector and in the hospital sub-sector and particularly at the CHUY of Yaounde. First category public hospitals like the CHUY are endowed with a legal personality and financial autonomy. As such, they are Public Administrative Establishments (EPA) to which are applied not only the public health legislation applicable to any other public structure, but also the specific laws and regulations (collective agreements for first category hospitals, staff status, internal regulations, etc.).

1.1.2. Scientific justification

On the scientific level, the literature of health law in general and health legislation in particular is not sufficiently developed in Cameroon. However, as science has evolved, so has technology, the need to adapt to the new requirements of globalization is necessary. According to Nkoum (2005), scientific research allows us to question our practices, our behaviors and our visions of things and leads to the discovery of certain facets of reality. Through this work, which focuses on the impact of health legislation on the management of Cameroonian hospitals, we will promote health law and encourage others to pay particular attention to this discipline in Cameroon. Furthermore, our objective is to highlight the impact of health legislation in the management of first category hospitals, in this case the University Hospital of Yaoundé, and to identify legislation likely to boost the development of these hospitals.

1.2. Context of the study

The health sector is undergoing major changes that require an adapted management response. The failures experienced in the management of the country's health facilities, particularly those of the first category, explain the need for a new management profile, in order to be able to accompany and manage the new hospital, health and social governance. As a result, management techniques have gradually been called upon to penetrate the hospital sector, as Drucker had already noted in 1984. The application of management techniques to the health sector results in changes in professional practices which, in turn, have an impact on the organization, structure and management of health care in general. It should be remembered that the definition of the hospital and its standards of execution are a function of the transformations that affect the mores, habits, values and culture of society (Ogrizek and Alii, 1996). In this respect, it is necessary to develop technical skills in management, management and law[3] , but also to respect legal standards, and even to ensure that hospital management complies with existing standards.In Cameroon, studies on the determination of the percentage of health facilities (FOSA) that apply the health legislation in force and specific to hospitals and health facilities are not sufficiently developed. Even if we note the absence of a better legal framework, Cameroon is a state governed by the rule of law that wants to see its institutions function according to the legislation in force. Clearly, the health facilities in Cameroon generally operate in a disorderly fashion to the detriment of the texts. existing legal frameworks[4]. This situation is observed in first category hospitals such as the University Hospital of Yaoundé. This tends to attenuate the effects of health legislation on the management of these hospitals.At the CHUY, the role played by the health legislation can be very considerable insofar as its absence or the lack of its application within this hospital establishment reflects the bad state of the said hospital and university center. Indeed, a careful reading of certain texts applicable to first category hospitals, to the personnel and employees in the said establishments shows a flagrant violation of the rules of law in force in Cameroon. This violation or disregard of the legal rules leads to bad governance which translates into misappropriation of public funds, financial embezzlement, violation of the rights and freedoms of patients, bad treatment even of users[5]. However, the hospital has a public mission and its goal is to improve the health of the population. As such, the patient is no longer considered as an ordinary client but as a patient who is entitled to all the special attention. As we often say, **"the customer is king"**.

In a context marked by the requirement of modernization of medical practices and rationalization of the management of the **"public thing"**, Cameroonian hospitals must adapt to this new world order. At the Yaounde University Hospital Center, the strikes that have been going on for several years are intensifying and continue to this day. This multiplication of strikes can be explained by the very treatment of the staff of this university health establishment. The most probable explanation is the violation of the legal provisions in force, notably the status of the personnel, the collective agreement of the first category hospitals. We can undoubtedly deduce that health legislation has an influence on the management of health facilities in Cameroon in general and mainly in first category hospitals such as CHU Y. The present study carried out at the Yaoundé University Hospital takes place in Cameroon in a context of generalized crisis, particularly financial, economic, social, etc. ...

1.3. Problem of the study

A problem is a break between everyday life and the norm. It arises either from a failure to comply with an obligation or from an action taken in defiance of certain rules established in society. In this case, the health legislation exists so that it can be put to good use in order to allow for better care of patients and to stimulate the growth of hospital and health structures. However, the functioning of our health facilities seems to remove all ambiguity and deviate from the norm. At the Yaoundé University Hospital Center (CHUY), the multiplication of strikes and demands from the staff show that there is a break between the equitable management of the resources available in this university hospital and the practice of "opaque management" (Ateba Eyene, 2010). The corollary is staff dissatisfaction. In addition, this situation, which persists at the Yaoundé University Hospital, seems to pose a problem of results-based management, which would be oriented towards respecting the legal rules in force in the health sector. However, there is an arsenal of legal rules whose respect can contribute to the improvement of the management of the country's hospitals, especially the CHUY.

1.4. Issue

According to Nkoum (2005), "to construct a problematic is to elaborate the main theoretical reference points of one's research (...) It is to explore the fundamental concepts and general ideas that will allow one to construct a framework of analysis. Thus, the hospital must be identified in its complex structure and functioning. Here. it gathers a plurality of actors in its heart who, most often maintain the conflictual relations. In order to regulate the relationships between these actors and to promote more effective management, health law, through its legislation, proposes to develop the legal framework of health facilities.Hospital and health management, as a discipline of management sciences must be based on transparency, mastery and knowledge of legal and socio-administrative texts. It is what will lead to managerial innovation in Cameroonian hospitals. As such, the respect of the norm is essential to any structure that wants to be organized and that must function to produce more satisfactory results. To be effective, hospital and health management is based on certain theories. For Fortin (1996), a theory is a "set of generalizations about concepts and variables, intended to explain and predict phenomena". This discipline takes into consideration many theories. In the context of our study, the human relations approach, the systemic approach and the pure theory of law will be the focus of our attention. Hospital work must be carried out in accordance with existing regulations, hence the notable intervention of health legislation in the Cameroonian hospital field in general, and in the Yaoundé University Hospital Center (CHUY) in particular. What about research questions?

1.5. Research Questions

In this section, we will identify the general issue of this theme and the specific issues.

1.5.1 The general question

The overall research question for this study is:

What is the impact of health legislation on the management of the Yaoundé University Hospital Center?

L5.2 Specific issues

Specific questions that arise from the general question are:
1. What is the current state of health legislation applicable in first category hospitals (case of CHU Y)?
2. How is health legislation applied at UHC?

3. What are the effects of the health legislation (as it is applied) in the management of the CHUY?

It is this set of questions that will guide our study at the Yaoundé University Hospital Center (CHUY).

1.6. Research objectives

The research objectives of this study are presented in two forms: the general objective and the specific objectives.

1.6.1 The general research objective

The overall objective of this research is to:

To analyze the impact of health legislation in the management of the Hospital and University Center.

1.6.2 Specific objectives

The specific research objectives of this study are:

1. To take **stock of the** health legislation applicable to first category hospitals in Cameroon and to highlight its capacity to allow the development of CHUY;
2. Describe the application of health legislation at UHC;

3. Determine the effects of health legislation in the management of CHUY.

1.7. Interests of the study

Durkheim (1960) wrote: "we believe that our research is not worth an hour's effort if it were to be of only speculative interest "6 . It is from this position that the research on the impact of health legislation in the management of the University Hospital Center is of interest insofar as it attempts to provide legal and managerial support to the first category hospital training in our country (through the study carried out at the CHUY). In this respect, our study presents personal, legal, scientific, professional and social issues.

1.7.1. Personal interest

On a personal level, this study allowed us to better understand the notions of "health legislation" and "health facility management" and to see the interactions that exist between these two notions. It also provided us with the legal tools for managing hospital and health structures and stimulated our desire to do research, which is a student and professional necessity. Finally, it allowed us to meet all the requirements for obtaining a Master's degree in Hospital and Health Management (MGHS) at the School of Health Sciences of the Catholic University of Central Africa (ESS/UCAC) in Yaoundé.

1.7.2. Legal and scientific interest

From a legal and scientific point of view, the study of the impact of health legislation on the management of the CHUY allows us to visit a field which, to our knowledge and through our investigations, has not yet been explored in our country. It is about the sanitary and hospital legislation, the relations that this one maintains with the hospital management still remain less thought. This study therefore makes it possible to bring out the legal aspects that concern health and hospital management that have been hidden or buried in extra-health and extra-hospital texts until now. The aim of the research being to produce new knowledge on reality, this study undoubtedly contributes to the improvement of the management of our hospital and health structures, to the knowledge of health legislation, its respect and its application at a time when Cameroonian hospitals require urgent managerial intervention.

1.7.3. Professional interest

The results of this study could be useful to hospital managers and enable them to review their management methods and techniques. In addition, this study will be of considerable use to lawyers and health professionals in that it will provide them with the material they need to manage hospitals in accordance with Cameroonian law.

1.7.4. Social interest

On the social level, our study will be able to make a significant contribution to the improvement of hospital management in Cameroon, which will allow for better care of patients and more efficient management of health conditions. Clearly, our study will allow for a better satisfaction of the population.

CHAPTER 2
THEORETICAL AND CONCEPTUAL FRAMEWORK OF THE STUDY

In this part, it is a question of finding the relevant documents, i.e. the books dealing with the theme approached in this study, specialized reviews and acts of scientific conferences in order to work out the various concepts which will enable us to support the analysis and the interpretation of the collected data.

2.1. Review of the literature

This first part of the second will allow us to review the writings of certain authors who have worked on health legislation and hospital management. In this respect, it will be necessary to present the previous works on health legislation before reviewing those on hospital management in particular.

2.1.1. Literature on health legislation

In Cameroon, health legislation has not been widely written. Nevertheless, there are many texts dealing with health issues. Therefore, we will first look at the work of certain authors and international bodies, and then at Cameroonian health legislation.

2.1.2. Review of the international health literature

The WHO is the main body in the world that sets health standards. Nowadays, there are about a hundred legal texts and documents that deal with health problems in the world. By the way, the WHO created a department of "Health Legislation" in 1948. The work of this department has allowed the continuous publication of the journal "International Compendium of Health Legislation", the most important of which is that of 1998.[7]Through this continuous publication, several articles have been published. There is also a bulletin of the "International Office of Public Hygiene". In addition, according to article 63 of the WHO Constitution[8]Each Member State shall promptly communicate to the Organization all important laws, regulations, official reports and statistics concerning health published in that State. This gives us reason to quote in this work any legal text related to health and POSA management. Fluss (1998), in an article entitled "The role of WHO in the field of health legislation: a historical overview", notes the importance and role of health legislation in the field of public health and the need for "information transfer and technical cooperation to meet the needs of Member States at all stages of their economic and social development, irrespective of their political and legal systems" and to enable the harmonious functioning of the health and hospital authorities in evidence in those States.For Roemer (1998), health legislation is not only an instrument of public health but also of health policy. In one article, he notes the importance of health legislation in that "legislation is the cornerstone of all public health activity. It ... provides the legal framework for health policy. Without legislation, a public health official would have limited powers to clean up the environment, control the spread of disease, or allocate funds to maternal and child health programs. Of course, voluntary organizations and

8

the private sector are involved in many ways in the development and promotion of health policy; (...)". In this respect, health legislation is a determining factor in the management of health services and particularly health facilities, whether public or private. The constitution of the World Health Organization (1948) recognized in its preamble that "governments have a responsibility for the health of their peoples, which they can meet only by taking appropriate health and social measures. According to Article 2 (f) of this Constitution, the Organization, in order to achieve its purpose, shall "To establish and maintain such administrative and technical services as may be necessary, including epidemiological and statistical services. These constitutional provisions of the WHO reflect the need for the Organization and the States to supervise public health in general and health services, in particular hospital services. The supervision by these authorities is a guarantee of good hospital governance synonymous with equitable hospital management. Cameroon seems to have played its part.

2.1.3. National health literature review

In Cameroon, there is a plethora of legal texts that deal with health issues. Unfortunately, these texts are not contained in a body of legal rules specific to public health and hospital management. However, in the course of this work, our research has enabled us to classify these texts according to the hierarchy of legal norms into two main categories: laws and regulations.With regard to the laws, the main one is Law No. 96/03 of January 4, 1996 on the Health Framework Law, which, according to Article 1, establishes the general framework for State action in the field of health, particularly through the national health policy. According to article 3 of this law, "the national health policy aims in particular
1. Integration of care at all levels of the system and consideration of priority programs and specific actions in all health facilities;
2. The rationalization of the management of infrastructures, equipment and personnel by the implementation of efficient information systems allowing a real planning which takes into account the assets, the needs and the objectives of the health service (...)
3. The promotion of centralized management of health services to involve communities and health professionals more in the financing and management of these services.
This legislative provision reflects the significant involvement of the State in the management of health and health structures. This state organization of health management is therefore possible thanks to the establishment of legal standards of supervision.
In addition, a law of the National Assembly N°2003/2006 of December 22, 2003 governs blood transfusion in Cameroon. This law has a considerable effect on the functioning of hospitals. Indeed, its application in our hospital services contributes to the promotion of patients' rights and to a better care of patients in our hospitals, which also contributes to the good management of these health facilities.
In addition to these two laws, we can cite Law No. 99/001 of April 7, 1999 on the practice and organization of the profession of optician, Laws No. 34 and 36 of August 10, 1990 on the practice and organization of the profession of physician in Cameroon and on t h e practice of the profession of dental surgeon, Law No. 88/022 of August 16, 1990 on the practice and organization of the profession December 1988 modifying the law n° 84/010 of December 5, 1984 fixing the organization of the medical-health professions: nurse, midwife and medical-health technician. This set of laws organizes the exercise of the health professions. In most of

these laws, no one can practice if he does not belong to the body. This measure allows to avoid clandestine personnel in the hospital, although those who exercise these professions by infraction are punished by the law.Law No. 74/18 of 5 December 1974 on the control of authorizing officers and managers of public funds and State enterprises, as amended by Law No. 76-4 of 8 July 1976, also deserves special attention. In fact, this text applies to Cameroonian public hospitals because, as already noted by Drucker (1984), management techniques have gradually been called upon to penetrate the hospital sector. In addition, for a more rational management of Cameroonian hospitals, it is all the more necessary to institute a control of the managers of public funds in a context marked by multiple abuses in financial management.From another perspective, Cameroon has a large number of sanitary regulations. In our study, we will limit ourselves to mentioning only a few of them. Let us first mention Decree N°2011/0004 of January 13, 2011, which sets out the modalities for the exercise of certain competencies transferred by the State to the communes in terms of the construction, equipment and management of District Medical Centers (CMA). Article 7, paragraph 1 of this decree states that "the commune participates in the management of the District Medical Centers, through the recruitment and provision of personnel as needed. Such a provision can only reinforce the contribution of the texts in the management of hospital structures in Cameroon.Moreover, the decrees n° 78/241 of June 24, 1978 and n° 91/065 of January 23, 1991 respectively on the creation and organization of a Hospital and University Center (CHU), organization of the Hospital and University Center of Yaoundé (CHUY) interest us because it directly concerns the structure which will house our study. In addition, we have decrees n° 63/DF/141 of 24 April 1963 fixing the tariffs for public health consultations, visits, deliveries, medical certificates as well as the value of the head letters of the nomenclature of professional acts, No. 68/DF/419 of 15 October 1968 to lay down the structural organization and organic functioning of hospital and health facilities in Cameroon, No. 92/252-PM of 6 July 1992 to lay down the conditions and modalities for the creation and opening of certain private health facilities, No. 92/226/PM of 22 July 1992 to lay down the modalities for the control of private health facilities, No. 92/226/PM of 22 July 1992 to lay down the modalities for the control of private health facilities. and n° 94/303/PM of June 14, 1994 fixing the modalities of the shares on the expensive transfers to certain medical and paramedical personnel practicing in the public medical formations. Following the decrees, we have the decree of September 20, 1999, modifying and completing certain provisions of the decree N° 05/MSP of July 15, 1994 fixing the modalities of internal allocation of the receipts intended for the expenses in the public health formations by decree N° 30/MSP dated September 20, 1999,the decree fixing the modalities of creation, organization and functioning of Health Districts by decree N°35-A-MSP-CAB dated October 8, 1999, the decree N° 631-CAB-PR dated December 3, 1987 on the classification of Private Health Facilities, the decree N° 15-MTPS-IMT dated October 15, 1979 fixing the modalities of organization and functioning of the occupational medical services Interministerial Order No. 1621/A/MSP/DS, No. 24/A/MINCI/DPPM sets the value of key letters corresponding to medical, surgical or specialist acts and medical analyses in the nomenclature of professional acts in the private health sector. Order No. 0001/A/MSP/CAB of November 16, 1994 specifies the powers of the management committees of public health facilities and finally, Order No. 0003/MSP/CAB of November 16, 1994 sets the terms and conditions for allocating quotas to certain medical and paramedical staff.

2.1.4. Importance and role of health legislation

Nyemb (2012) defined health legislation as "the body of laws and regulations that govern health matters. Health legislation plays a crucial role in the organization and functioning of a country, structure, organization or service. In an article, Liguerre states: "legislation and the range of existing standards constitute a set of performance requirements stated in a prescriptive manner and available to all". For this author, legislation is a guarantee of an organization's performance. In the same vein, Owona (2013), welcoming the work conducted by Ondoa (2013), stated that many leaders make bad decisions because they are not aware of the legal texts in force in our country. These statements show the importance of legislation in the organization and functioning of a structure or organization such as a hospital. Legislation taken as a set of legal texts allows, through laws, regulations and many others, to establish uniform standards intended for the regulation of human activity, the behavior of the latter and even its ways of doing in a given society. As such, it is very often taken in the form of a law that enacts rules to be followed and whose violation is sanctioned by an organ, usually the judiciary.

2.2. The literature on hospital management

This first part of our study allowed us to visit the publications of many authors on hospital management. Thus, in a book entitled "Hospital Management: A Handbook of Hospital Governance and Law", Holcman (2015) believes that the new governance requires its actors to master the rules of management of health care institutions (public or private) in a constantly changing context. The author sets out to meet this need in this book, which covers almost all aspects of hospital law: public hospital service, planning, external and internal governance, quality of care, health safety, liability, ethics and patients' rights, and professional conduct. It also provides the keys to understanding hospital management: T2A, cost accounting, EPRD, public procurement, PMS1, performance, work organization, demographic perspectives, GPEC.Similarly. Nobre and Lambert (2012) consider that the reorganization of the governance of health care institutions has a restructuring effect on the role and positioning of the players. The unit is now the basic management unit and the place where medical strategy is implemented. The cluster contract, which defines the scope and terms of management delegation, has become the preferred tool for internal management. This book should therefore be used as a reference manual for the training of management teams and executives in health care institutions.Faced with the growing complexity of health care institutions, Hart and Sylvie (2002) agree in "Management hospitalier: Stratégies nouvelles des cadres" that there is an urgent need to define the contours of hospital management. Through this book, the two authors make the social sciences accessible to change the way health managers and their partners look at their work context. Their ambition is t o inscribe managers in a new posture that opens them t o other possibilities. These The authors therefore stipulate that by developing their strategic intelligence both towards the services for which they are responsible and towards their partners who form the basis of their relational fabric, health managers can find opportunities in change projects to anchor new practices in the major current institutional orientations."Executives, operational executives, managers and administrators in a private or public health care institution, you are faced with the same challenge every day: to combine the quality of care and the quality of life at work of your employees, all in a context of permanent rationalization of means" Benoit (2015: 38). To solve this delicate equation of **combining quality of care and quality of work life,** the author believes that it is necessary to revisit organizational modes, management practices and dare to apply new management tools that include respect for health standards.

2.2.1. The relationship between health legislation and hospital management

In general, management aims to increase the competitiveness, performance and image of an organization. To this end, it employs numerous material, financial and human resources. In an environment as delicate as that of the hospital, marked on the one hand by the need for better care of patients and the needy, and on the other hand by the requirements of job security and revenue, health legislation acts as a guide, a line, a course of action to be followed in order to achieve such an approach. The review of the literature that we have just presented above leads us to a conceptual elaboration.

2.3. Conceptual development

A concept is "a word or set of words that designates a set of real phenomena" (Nkoum, 2005: 78). Generally speaking and from a theoretical point of view, concepts define, according to the same author, what the researcher intends to observe on the basis of empirical tests. For Valider Marren (2000: 12) "a concept must be defined according to the field in which it will be used, in order to avoid confusion of meaning linked to the polysemy of the said concepts". Thus, it is necessary to agree on the key terms used, in order to make our research topic more understandable. It These are mainly incidence, health legislation, management.

2.3.1. The impact

According to the Dictionnaire Encyclopédique de Langue Française (1996), incidence refers to the more or less direct consequence of something; a repercussion. Impact can be positive or negative. It is positive when it brings about positive results or enables a good action to be carried out, in other words, when it has a positive impact. On the other hand, it is negative when it negatively influences a fact.

2.3.2. Sanitary

For the Petit Larousse illustré of 2012, the adjective sanitary refers to anything related to the preservation of public health. It is in this sense, we speak of "sanitary regulation". 11 also refers to what is related to the facilities and equipment for the care of cleanliness, hygiene. This is the case of sanitary equipment such as incubators, medical analysis equipment, etc.

2.3.3. Health legislation

Etymologically, the word "legislation" comes from the Latin legislatio, which designates the law itself, from lex, legis, which also means "written law". It has often designated the science of the knowledge of laws. This is why we speak of "courses in legislation".In a broad sense, legislation refers to all the laws and regulations of a country, legislative provisions concerning a particular field: Cameroonian legislation, labor legislation. As such, it includes the constitution, the laws enacted by the legislative power, i.e. the parliament, the administrative regulations emanating from the executive power, i.e. the decrees, the orders and, to a certain extent, the circulars which apply in a specific field[9]. Thus, health legislation would then be "a set of laws and regulations that govern health matters" as Nyemb (2012) well presents it.Health legislation may be general or specific. It is general when it applies to all areas or to a set of activities, establishments or to several sectors of activity such as health, transport, trade, industry, etc... In this respect, we can mention the finance law, the presidential decree of 12 December 1999 on the general status of Public Administrative Establishments (EPA), Public and Parapublic Companies. On the other hand, it is specific when it applies exclusively to a particular field or service. This is the case of Law N° 2003/2006 of 22 December 2003 governing blood transfusion in Cameroon.

> **The different components of health legislation**

The word "legislation" was once the name given to the power granted to certain authorities to issue binding rules. Nowadays, it is generally used to refer to the body of laws and regulations in force in a given state. One will speak for example of the Cameroonian legislation. Similarly, in a less general sense, the word "legislation" can be used to restrict its scope to a specific subject. In this sense, one might say "refer to the legislation on divorce". As we have already pointed out, legislation includes the Constitution, the rules laid down by Parliament, i.e. the National Assembly and the Senate, administrative regulations such as decrees, orders and, to a certain extent, circulars.

- The constitution

The constitution is the fundamental and supreme norm in a state. It defines fundamental rights, determines the organization of public powers and the relations between them and, through organic laws, structures the institutions of the Republic. In Cameroon, there is a constitutional silence with regard to the enactment of health standards. The constitutional law of January 18, 1996 does not therefore expressly provide for provisions relating to health.

- Rules set by parliament: the law

In the broadest sense, a law is a normative and abstract provision laying down a legal rule of mandatory application. The rule of law is a tool at the disposal of the citizen that allows him to render a work in conformity with the ideal of justice. It is in this sense that laws n° 96/03 of January 4, 1996 on the Framework Law in the field of Health and n° 34 and 36 of August 10, 1990 on the practice and organization of the profession of physician in Cameroon and on the practice of the profession of dental surgeon, respectively, are adopted. In addition, any freedom or any right necessarily implies, in order to be exercised completely, a duty of tolerance and respect, even of responsibility. In the formal sense, a law is a provision made by a deliberation of Parliament, as opposed to a regulation, which is issued by one of the administrative authorities to which the constitutional laws have conferred regulatory power. It is then a written rule of a permanent nature with a general scope and an imperative character, elaborated and voted by an elected parliament, promulgated by the President of the Republic and published in the official gazette in French and English, in the case of Cameroon. In Cameroon, there is a small volume of legislative texts (laws) in the area of health, but a predominance of regulatory texts.

- Administrative acts or regulations

An administrative act is a legal act made within the framework of the administration and in the general interest. It is precisely an act taken by the administration creating rights and obligations towards the citizens. The administrative act must be in conformity with a set of rules of law which form the administrative legality. There are two types of administrative acts: unilateral administrative acts and administrative contracts. In our study, only the first type will be considered.The Cameroonian administrative judge, in the 1968 Ngongang Ndjanke case[10]defines a unilateral administrative act as a unilateral legal act taken by an administrative authority in the exercise of an administrative power and creating rights and obligations for individuals. It is presumed to be legal as long as a judge has not declared it illegal and is imposed on its recipients without their consent, because of the privilege of prior consent enjoyed by the administration (Mballa Owona, 2011: 74). It is therefore an act that creates law that can be referred to the judge of excess of power for censure in order to obtain its cancellation. A distinction is then made between non-enforceable acts or acts without grievance and enforceable acts or acts with grievance.A unilateral administrative act that is not enforceable or not grievable is an administrative act that is not subject to appeal. In this type of administrative act unilateral acts, circulars are in the second category and directives constitute a third category of acts that cannot be grieved.

The unilateral administrative acts that are enforceable or have a grievance are administrative acts that can be appealed. A distinction is made between regulatory acts which define a general situation, non-regulatory acts which consist mainly of individual decisions, i.e. characterizing an individual situation, collective decisions concerning several persons whose situation is interdependent and particular decisions for individualized situations which have effects on an indeterminate number of persons. Examples:

- regulations: prohibition of visits during working hours, working hours;

- individual decision: the appointment of the Director General of the CHUY or of a department head;

- collective decision: the compulsory wearing of gowns for the nursing staff;

- specific decision: declaration of public utility.

The distinction is not made on the number of recipients but on the individualization of this decision. This distinction is not absolute, so some acts can be both. Moreover, some acts are subject to a legal regime that borrows from both categories.

If the validity, i.e. the legal regularity of an administrative act is assessed as soon as it is signed, its opposability, i.e. its capacity to produce legal effects with regard to persons, is assessed only once these addressees have been informed by an adequate publicity. For regulatory acts, enforceability is subject to publication, posting of the act or any other written means, not including telephone messages. Thus, decrees must be published in the Official Gazette as well as laws and the constitution.

> **The role of health legislation**

Health facilities provide a public service and are largely responsible for promoting and restoring the health of individuals. As such, they deserve to be provided with a clear legal basis, resources and a structured intervention program leading to the rationalization of their organization and treatment.Health legislation is an inseparable and primary part of any policy for the management of hospital structures, which, for a country, is realized in a national health policy. In the same way that it is normal to have policies in the field of Because of its ever-increasing impact on the practice of health management, legislation represents an important and complex field of study and reflection, whether it be economic development, the environment, education, culture or leisure. It is important because the solution to most of the difficulties encountered by hospital management lies mainly in the legislative infrastructure (Couture & Lajeunesse, 1991: 426).Even today, several countries have not established a legal reference in the field of health and see these as general provisions, for example, in the protection of cultural heritage, historical monuments and archaeological discoveries, when it is not simply administrative law.However, it is essential to have more specific legal and administrative texts on the organization of hospital management. Without these texts, health systems and services with any chance of success cannot be created and, above all, cannot exist. The lack of a solid legal basis aggravates the misunderstanding of management.

> **The nature and character of legislation as a rule of law**

Legislative rules are rules of law. A rule of law is a rule of conduct, a commandment that must allow a collective life, as harmonious as possible. It generally has three (3) characteristics. Thus, it must be general, abstract and mandatory. In this sense, legislation can be general in scope when it governs a specific case, i.e. a situation that can be applied in a series of concrete cases or that pursues a goal of general interest.The rule of law is abstract when it is not aimed at a particular person. It must be aimed at an abstract group of people. In this case, it is said to be impartial, impersonal and binding on all. This is where the maxim **"no one is above the law"** comes from. The General Statute of the EPA is a good illustration of this. However, a derogation f r o m this point is allowed. Thus, certain rules of law can be specific, i.e. they can pursue a particular interest. In this derogatory case, it is individual and does not concern everyone. This is the case of the act or decree appointing the Director General of the CHUY. Finally, the rule of law has a binding force. Because it gives a general order, any person who does not respect it can be forced to do so or sanctioned. It is this constraint that gives it its primacy.

2.3.4. Management

By management we mean a set of techniques for directing, organizing and managing a company11. According to Alison (1993), management is "the organization and direction of resources in order to achieve a desired result. In a broader sense, Thiétard defines it as an operational perspective, the action or fart of leading an organization, directing it, planning its growth and development, and controlling it. It is also the set of leaders of a company. For Ateba Eyene (2010), "the English verb <- manage" and the term "management" come from the

French word "ménager" meaning the action of regulating well, of disposing well: it is the art of leading and directing". The same author adds "management is defined as all the techniques of organization and management of 1 company to lead, to direct the action of the individuals". If managing is organizing, directing a company, a service, then hospital management would be the art of organizing, leading and managing hospitals, these being the establishments, public or private, where medical or surgical care is provided12.For Drucker (1984), management is "the activity of obtaining a collective result from people by giving them a common goal, common values, a suitable organization and the necessary training so that they perform well and adapt to change. As such, every manager's mission is to implement the technical, financial and human means to achieve his objectives.Crener and Monteil (1979), speaking of management, write: "from a rigorous knowledge of economic, social and human facts and of the opportunities offered by the environment (market, economic policy), management is a way of rationally directing and managing an organization (company, public body, association), of organizing activities, of setting goals and objectives, of building strategies. It will achieve this by making the best use of people, material resources, machines and technology, with the aim of increasing the profitability and efficiency of the company. If we want to To update this definition, it will be necessary to integrate the organization's capacity to anticipate the evolution of all its environments. This collection of definitions clearly shows the broadening of the field of study. It is a question of looking at the organizational phenomenon as a whole, which includes all possible forms of management that can be applied to a hospital establishment. The management of these structures essentially concerns the problems of coordination and management of internal resources, and not only the allocation of these resources.

> **Management styles**

There is no ideal reference, the effectiveness or ineffectiveness of a management style depends on the situation encountered and the state of mind of the employees, their maturity. The management style can also be a function of the type of organization, the size of a company, and the personality of the leader(s), as we have already pointed out. Thus the size of the company, the sector of activity, the structure of the managing company (family or not) and the structure of the organization (centralized or decentralized hierarchy) also influence management styles (Mintzberg, 1984). There are four main management styles. Of course, a person is never entirely one or the other of these models, except in pathological cases. Depending on the situation or even on the mood of the moment, the manager uses this or that style of management and then another without being locked into a single way of being and doing. These four main management styles are :

⁜ Participative management

Associating and involving are the key words of participative management (Chatenay, 2012). This management style is based on relational qualities and proposes to involve the personnel in the decision-making process in a logic of delegation of power. It aims to improve the working conditions of the staff, and therefore, the production through a real team collaboration.

Table 1: Summary of participative management

	Interests	Limits
The line manager	he shows his "support", his defense of the team's interests	Decision-making is slow. Lack of authority can lead to conflict within the team of the team
The collaborators	The interest shown by the responsible for individuals	Insecurity born of shared problems

Sources: Chateiiay (2012), Fiches pratiques management 2 - 5

+ Persuasive management

Its key word is "mobilize". This is a form of management where collective cohesion is paramount. In this style of management, the manager must listen to the members of the organization, create links between them while knowing how to make effective decisions quickly. It is a management model that requires both organizational and relational qualities.

Table 2: Summary of persuasive management

	Interests	Limits
The line manager	The exemplary nature of the "leader" is a source of energy and collective learning	The energy required and the risk of exhaustion
The collaborators	(if the style is adapted) The development of the relationship between the leader and his team	(If the style is not adapted) The prevention of the affirmation of the abilities of the employees

Sources: Chatenay, Practical management sheets 2 - 4

+ **Delegative management**

The objective of the delegative style is to give responsibility to the agents or collaborators, i.e. to leave the hands free to the personnel so that they can regulate themselves and take responsibility for themselves. 11 is based on the manager's total trust in his team. In this case, the autonomy and freedom of initiative offered to the staff increase their motivation and performance.

17

Table 3: Summary of delegative management

	Interests	Limits
The line manager	Time saving and possibility to invest in missions particular	Fear of uselessness and loss of control of the person in charge
The collaborators	Maximum accountability of agents	(if the style does not match) Work inefficiency and disorder

Sources: Chatenay, Practical management sheets 2 - 6

🞣 Directive management

Structure is the main characteristic of directive management. This style of management is based on an organization established beforehand and imposed on the staff. Decision-making is the responsibility of the manager who positions himself as a superior, expert and entitled to demand an immediate and effective response from his team. This style of management would be the one adopted by the University Hospital of Yaoundé. However, it is not impossible that the manager or director delegates part of his or her authority and skills to an agent to perform a specific task.

Besides these four management styles, there are several forms of management. These include:

- **Organizational management,** which includes the fields of production of goods and services, communication, marketing, human resources (HR) and financial and budgetary policies;

- **Operational management,** which refers to all the managerial techniques implemented for the administration of an organization;

- **Strategic management** which concerns the general directions and orientations adapted by the company according to the organization and the market environment;

- **Project management,** which allows you to organize a project from start to finish and ensure its success;

- **Marketing management,** which is generally based on a market study to analyze the needs and behaviors of consumers;

- **quality management,** which aims to improve the quality of an organization's services or products; etc.

➢ **The management process**

Management is based on four (4) main activities: planning, organizing, directing and controlling. Health care institutions are nowadays confronted with a double constraint, a strong growth in the qualitative and quantitative requirements concerning their services and, at the same time, a strengthening of budgetary constraints (Nobre, 2001: 129)[13].

2.3.5. University Hospital Center (CHU)

A University Hospital is a hospital establishment in which care is provided by senior health professionals and students. A UHC is usually linked to a university. Students do their practical teaching in the UHC on real patients. The teaching concerns general or specialized medicine, paramedical professions and science researchers.

In Cameroon, there is only one UHC classified as a first category hospital. This is the University Hospital of Yaoundé which serves as the setting for this study. This hospital has several objectives, namely to provide care, conduct research, support academic programs and cooperation. Because of its dual status of care and training, the management of the CHU is efficient, rational and better equipped than that of a simple hospital establishment and that of a university because it is neither one nor the other, but both at the same time.

2.4. Conceptual diagram

The conceptual scheme reflects the thematic flow of our field of investigation. Thus, the figure presented below represents the conceptual scheme of our study.

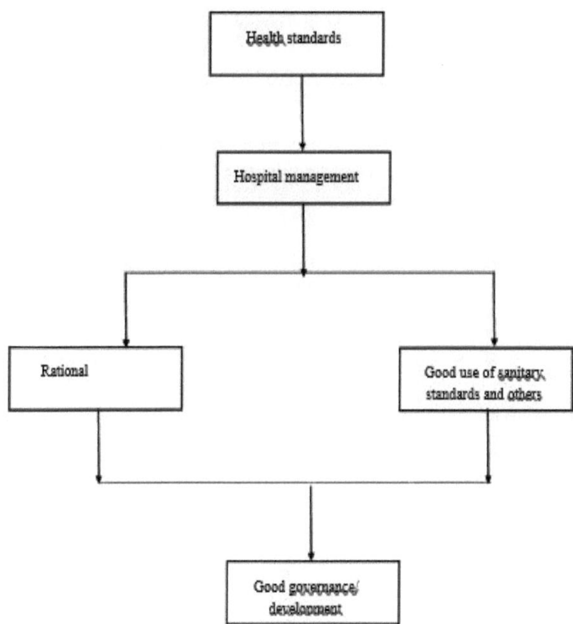

➢ **Explanation of the conceptual diagram**

The diagram above highlights the link between health standards and hospital management. With regard to legal norms, as we have emphasized above, they are a set of Laws and Regulations in force in a given State and include the Constitution, the rules set by Parliament, i.e. the National Assembly and the Senate, and administrative regulations such as decrees, orders and, to a certain extent, circulars, which apply to the health sector. Legal norms are then intended to regulate, or at least organize, a given sector. In our case, health standards have an influence on managerial practiceshospital management. The health standard or legislation therefore organizes hospital management to a significant degree.Management, as Ateba Eyene (2010) has so well noted, seeks "effectiveness and efficiency in (...) managing the knowledge of all actors, while exercising a certain degree of power and direction". It is a way of federating all energies for the materialization of programmed objectives. In this perspective, hospital management or managing a hospital structure means promoting more rational, more effective and more efficient management of this hospital training. For our study, health legislation organizes hospital management, which promotes the rational management of hospital structures. Rational management, it seems to me, is a factor in the good governance of health structures.Every society seeks the well-being of its people. By well-being, we mean the idea of satisfying human needs, whether personal or common. When hospital facilities in a country are well managed, i.e. when the objectives defined by hospital establishments are effectively achieved, we can speak of good hospital governance. Sound management is at the same level as compliance with the norm. Compliance with the standard and rational management of the UHC Y can lead to good governance of health care institutions. Good hospital governance is at a strategic level, as is the rational management of an institution, in the sense that it concerns both the management itself, compliance with the law and the structural organization that enables this management to be implemented. To sum up, health regulation or legislation is of capital interest for good hospital governance in developing countries like ours.

Table 5: Analysis Model

Concepts	Dimension	Components	Indicators
Incidence	Positive Negative	Rational organization, predefined results Disorder, claims, uprisings, strikes	Efficiency
			Efficiency
			The chaos
			Results not achieved
Health legislation	Legal Regulatory	Laws Decrees, orders, circulars, memos	General guidelines
			Implementation of Policies
			Compliance with the standard
Hospital management	Human Resources Management	GPEC	Recruiting
			Mobilization
			Evaluation
			Training
			Departures
	Management of Material Resources	Administrative materials	Furniture
		Technical equipment	Consumables medical and drugs
	Financial Resources Management	Revenues Expenditures	Budgeting
			Financing
			Securing funds
			Disbursement of funds
			Use of funds

According to Fortin (1996), a theory is a "set of generalizations concerning concepts and propositions specifying relations between variables, intended to explain and predict phenomena. It is therefore a system of abstract concepts which, to quote Nkoum (2005), attempts to explain and rationalize the world. In the field of management, several theories and models have been developed with the aim of improving the efficiency and effectiveness of organizations. As an organization, the hospital has inherited several of these theories that will contribute to the theoretical framework and conceptual models of our study.

2.5.1. Presentation of the theory

According to Dépelleau (2000), the choice of a theory depends above all on its relevance to the reality under study, i.e., the one that seems to correspond best to the reality being studied. For Nkoum (2005), "a theoretical framework is a set of knowledge, concepts, theories, and references that make it possible to describe, explain, and analyze the research question or the hypothesis stated.In the field of management, there is a multiplicity of schools that develop a multitude of theories. Among these multiple schools we can mention the Classical School, the School of Human Relations, the School of Contingency, the Sociological School, the Knowledge Management and the Professionals. Within the framework of our work, the pure theory of law and the theory of organizations, with the classical school, have retained our attention.

2.5.2. Hans Kelsen's Pure Theory of Law

Taking up and summarizing the essential theses of his theory. Kelsen (1934) wants to show the requirement of specificity of any theory of law in relation to the natural sciences based on the principle of causality as well as in relation to ethics and politics. For the author, it is possible to systematically describe a certain legal order or to present a defined group of norms of such an order or to highlight a particular regulation. In this way, Kelsen (1934) considers that one can try to clarify the norms under consideration or the regulation in question, to specify their meaning as it immediately results from the authentic formulation that the law adopts in the form of a law, a decree, a regulation, etc. In this perspective, the description of the law is linked to its interpretation. According to Fauteur, it is also possible to compare the contents of different legal orders in order to identify certain legal types. Finally, on the basis of a comparison of all the phenomena considered as belonging to the law, one can also search for its essence, its proper structure and this independently of the material changes it adopts in time and space. It must determine the specific method and the fundamental concepts and provide the theoretical foundations for any analysis relating to a particular law or to particular legal institutions. The pure theory of law intends to be this general theory. As a theory proposing a specific method of knowledge of law, it submits to a logical analysis the propositions with which this science describes its object. In other words, clic establishes the conditions of possibility of the statements concerning obligations, rights, responsibility, subjects of law, physical and moral persons, organs, and competence. By this means, it arrives at the central concept of all legal knowledge, the concept of norm, which expresses the idea that a certain human behavior must be subject to precise conditions and searches, within the hypothetical judgments that characterize the legal propositions, for the specific meaning scion which a condition is linked to its consequence. This theory, which has given rise to a very famous current in law, namely legal positivism, is largely useful to us in the analysis of our data. Legal positivism is a current that describes the law as it exists in society, rather than as it should be, and consists of rejecting the importance of an ideal law and affirming that only positive law, i.e. laws and jurisprudence, has a legal value. Thus, the law or jurisprudence would be the only norm to be respected (legalist positivism). The fundamental problem of the positivists consists therefore in the multiplicity of legislations, the law in force in a given country changes in time and space. He elaborates a theory of law which allows to find the common element to all positive rights. He establishes, first of all, that all positive rights contain legal norms. He then notes that their specificity in relation to other norms, social or moral, lies in the empowerment they receive from an authority. The judgment of a court is valid if it applies a law, thus a norm of a higher level. A positive legal system is therefore not defined by its different elements, but by its capacity to enforce this norm. This is the birth of another aspect of the pure theory of law, the hierarchy of legal norms. The notion of a hierarchy of norms was also formulated by the legal theorist Kelsen. According to him, every legal norm receives its validity from its conformity to a higher norm, thus forming a hierarchical order. The more important they are, the less the norms are numerous: the superposition of norms, i.e. circulars, regulations, laws, Constitution, thus acquires a pyramidal form, which explains why this theory is called pyramid of norms. In our analysis, this theory will allow us to verify the conformity of the acts taken at the CHUY.

2.5.3. Weberian theory: bureaucratic organization

Developed by Wcber (1992) in the Classical School[14]The theory of bureaucratic organization is intended to be a rational mode of organization, based on law and regulations, which must break with the arbitrariness and "a peu près" of the working world of the time. This traditional model legitimizes the authority of the chief through the belief in the inviolable nature of the administrative routine and the certainty of the predictability of the reactions of all the elements of the system. The fact that procedures are written down avoids any ambiguity in their implementation. Management exercises its authority through memos that immediately acquire legal force. For Weber (1992), this gives absolute objectivity to the decision-making process, gives the organization complete independence from political power, and at the same time sets a disciplinary framework. Analyzing the sources of power in three types of organizations, the German sociologist and lawyer presents the following properties of the bureaucratic organization: the hierarchical structure and the competences of each job are clearly defined, the remuneration is fixed and depends on the responsibilities and the hierarchical level, the discipline is strict, a separation exists between the job and the person who is not the owner of his or her position, written rules anticipate all situations, and the promotion is determined by the superior. Weber's work seems to emphasize the organization of work and the establishment of norms that should govern the functioning of a company[15]. He then presents four main principles of rational bureaucracy, namely :

➢ The division of labor which aims at increasing productivity;
➢ The hierarchical structure that determines the different levels of authority in an organization, the routing of information, the role played by each of its members;

➢ Vertical communication, which consists of circulating information in a hierarchical manner, i.e. from the top down;
➢ Written information consisting of memos, rules and procedures established in writing to avoid misinterpretation.

Like the pure theory of law, the theory of bureaucratic organization led the analysis of the results of our study in the sense that it allowed us to analyze the organization and functioning, as well as the sources of power and the conformity of the texts taken at the CHUY in relation to the existing norms.

2.5.4 The theory of the Administrative Function

The theory of the administrative function was developed in the classical school by Fayol (1916). According to this author, to administer is to foresee, to organize, in the strong sense of the term, to constitute the organism that is the company. It is also to command, that is to say to allow the personnel to fulfill their functions by giving them orders. It also means coordinating and harmonizing the efforts and work of each person in a group. Finally, it is to control, to see to the respect of the established orders and rules. These are the five administrative functions, it being understood that one should not confuse "governing", which is to ensure the best functioning of the organization in the essential operations mentioned above, and "administering", which corresponds more specifically to the last of these. It is Fayol who insisted on the need for organizational leaders to acquire administrative training, or even management training. According to Daval (2015), Fayol's theory of Administrative Function is not only a science of work, it deals with human organization, which no longer has as its sole end performance, but the best overall functioning of the company, and which, therefore, concerns leaders more than executors. It is a question of rationalizing such a set. To this end, it is essential to draw up "organization charts" that allow one to grasp at a glance the entire organization, the departments, their structures and the hierarchical chain. It is through the meticulous study of these charts, the ancestors of what we now call the organization chart, that we will discover all the defects of organization, or that we will detect the absence of unity in command, which constitutes the most serious fault in Fayol's eyes. In this perspective, this theory will help us to analyze, or even to take a look at the organizational chart of UHC to highlight the shortcomings or incongruities of the system. In addition, Fayol identified fourteen principles of administration. Among the most significant, the principle of authority is posited as "the right to command and the power to be obeyed". It is in this sense that Barnard (1976) showed that an unacknowledged authority is not an authority. Again announcing Barnard, Fayol adds that authority is inconceivable without responsibility, that is, without a sanction, a reward or a penalty, which accompanies the exercise of power.

2.5.5 The theory of modeling relationships within an organization

Mintzberg, in 1984[16] exposes the POPDCORB[17] developed by Gulick and Urwick (1937) and formed by the initials of the different management activities: Planning, Organization, Personnel, Direction, Coordination, Reporting and Budgeting. According to this author, POPDCORB also permeates the writings of successful theorists such as Drucker (1984), and those of business leaders like Ralph Cordiner. According to this theory, the effectiveness of an organization depends on the combination of these different management activities. Legislation intervenes in all these areas of activity either to organize them or to regulate them. In this respect, in this work which concerns the incidence of health legislation in the management of the University Hospital Center of Yaoundé, the theories previously mentioned will be of capital importance because they will allow us to better orient our study and to better elucidate our argument because as much as planning is important for the management of a structure such as the CHUY, it also requires a text, a regulation or a legislation

2.5.6 The use of theories

In this study, we used four theories to guide the analysis of our results. The pure theory of law, developed by Kelsen (1934), allowed us to analyze the codification and the conformity of the texts taken by the administration of the CHUY to the established higher legal norms. Weber's theory of bureaucratic organization (1992) This study allowed us to take a look at the organization of work at the CHUY and to analyze interpersonal communication, as well as the hierarchical structure of the center. The theory of the administrative function developed by Fayol (1916) was used in our study to analyze the management, its style and its components at the CHUY. Finally, the theory of modeling relationships within the administration allowed us to analyze the main activities carried out at the CHUY, their proper execution and the interactions that exist between the personnel in carrying out these activities.

CHAPTER 3
METHODOLOGICAL APPROACH TO THE STUDY

In a book on research methodology, it is stated that the population or parent population is the set of all individuals or groups of individuals with specific characteristics related to the objectives of the survey (Nkoum, 2005). As such, no study is possible unless the researcher circumscribes it within a given framework. Thus, our study, which will focus on the impact of health legislation on management, will be conducted at the Yaoundé University Hospital Center, which deserves to be presented in this chapter before addressing the methodological approach of our study.

3.1. Presentation of the study site

As we have just noted in previous lines, our study took place at the University Hospital Center of Yaoundé (CHUY). The choice of this site is justified by the mission of student supervision and research that the CHUY must promote. In addition, the many complaints and claims of the staff of this institution[18] have aroused in us the desire to conduct a study in these places.

3.1.1. History of CHUY

The CHUY is a Public Administrative Institution (EPA) with legal personality and financial autonomy. It is placed under the technical supervision of the Ministry of Public Health and under the financial supervision of the Ministry of Finance.The history of medical training in Cameroon begins with the setting up in 1965 of a commission led by Dr. Tsoungui and charged with the elaboration of the construction, operation and teaching program of the mixed faculty of medicine and pharmacy in Yaoundé[19]. The setting up of this commission was inspired by the observations of the conference of deans of the faculty of medicine of black Africa who found the western programs not adapted for doctors practicing in Africa. Given the relevance and the [18]We refer to the multiple strike calls made by the staff in the media since 2010.At stake in this project, the UNDP, in association with the WHO and other operators, has undertaken to pilot and finance a project to train doctors who should revolutionize medicine in Africa.[20]

Thus, in 1969, the first class of medical students entered the University Center for Health Sciences (CUSS) of Yaoundé. A few years later, with the creation of the CHUY in 1978, a new era opened up for the health services of medical students at CUSS. Between 1978 and 1988, the CHUY, set up as a reference hospital, had its moments of glory thanks to the performance of its administrative, financial and organizational management and the quality of its medical-technical services with its unique technical platform in Cameroon.

3.1.2 Geographic location of CHUY

The CHUY has its headquarters in Yaoundé, capital of the Republic of Cameroon. It is located in the department of Mfoundi, district of Yaoundé 3rd in the Melen district. Bounded on the East by the Faculty of Medicine and Biomedical Sciences (FMSB), on the West by the Polytechnic, passing by the EMIA crossroads, CHUY is to the South of the African Synergy and Suffering and to the North of the CIRCB.

3.1.3 CHUY's missions

UHC's mission is:
- The mission of providing high level medical and paramedical care

- The mission of pedagogical support to the training provided at the Faculty of Medicine and Biomedical Sciences (FMSB) of the University of Yaoundé T and in other training institutions in medical and paramedical care;
- The mission of promoting research in the health sciences;
- The mission of collaboration and cooperation with direct or indirect participation in all activities or operations of a scientific nature, in the health or medical field.

3.1.4 Organization of the CHUY

The operation of the CHUY is organized around :
➢ **At the strategic level,** there is the Board of Directors, which is the deliberative body that approves the major decisions concerning the Center, and the General Management, which is responsible for implementing the decisions and policies of operation and development
➢ **At the organizational level,** it includes the technical and medical management, the divisions and the departments
➢ **At the operational level,** a team composed of Doctors, aggregated or holders o f a

Doctorate in the different fields of medicine, academics, medical personnel in health care21 and Nurses, specialized or not,
In addition to these bodies, there are committees such as the Therapeutic Committee, the HIV'AIDS Comprehensive Care Committee, the Ethics Committee, the Hygiene Committee and the Blood Exposure Accident Committee, etc. The organizational chart in the appendix is of great importance in understanding the organizational structure of the CHUY.

3.1.5 Human Resources Management (HRM) at UHC

The staff of the CHUY is made up of 24 university hospitalists, 31 hospital practitioners, 9 general practitioners and 240 medical health personnel. It receives an average of 70 national and international residents and 216 students from the Faculty of Medicine and Biomedical Science of the University of Yaoundé I.

There are two types of personnel at the CHUY: civil servants and contract workers. The majority of the staff are contractual, i.e., recruited on the basis of an employment contract in accordance with Law No. 92/007 of August 14, 1992 on the Cameroonian Labor Code. Civil servants, who are in the minority, are assigned to the CHUY by the Ministry in charge of the civil service in collaboration with the Ministry of Health. However, it should be noted that this difference in status is not felt in this public administrative establishment, because the very status of these establishments excludes all personnel working in the EPAs. With regard to recruitment techniques, the procedures seem to be less well known. Moreover, an analysis of personnel needs is difficult to do in these places. According to a staff member we met at the CHUY personnel department, "there is no call for job offers and we are sometimes surprised to see an unknown individual arrive with a certificate of employment. Continuous training and retraining of personnel seem to be provided in this health facility. Internal mobility is carried out at the level of the general management and the personnel department. However, there is no planning for staff mobility, which sometimes results in an agent being transferred or unstable within one or two months.There are some problems with retirement. The age pyramid does not exist, which explains the presence in certain services of people who are close to or have reached the age of 70. Some employees do not benefit from their full rights. For example, in August, a dozen retired agents won their case after a lawsuit against the CHUY.With regard to staff motivation, the problem is acute at UHC. According to Besseyre et al (2008), motivation is "a force that pushes the individual to satisfy his or her needs, desires, and impulses, and that determines a behavior aimed at reducing a state of tension and thus restoring balance. However, order n°003/MSP/SAB of November 16, 1994 sets out the terms and conditions for the allocation of quotas to certain medical and paramedical personnel working in public health facilities. This decree seems to have no effect at the CHUY.

3.1.6. Management of Material and Financial Resources

The Yaounde University Hospital Center is endowed with twelve (12) validating university hospital services headed by professors of magisterial rank, lecturers, etc. It has many material and financial resources.With respect to material resources, there are movable and immovable assets and consumable goods under the management of the CHUY. Thus, this health facility has a capacity of 227 beds and in 2003 received 62,657 patients for consultation and 9957 for hospitalization, with a bed occupancy rate of around 80%. Formerly equipped with a technical platform at the cutting edge of a The CHUY remains a shadow of its former self, as its technical facilities have deteriorated[22].

Consumables are managed in each unit or department by the managers. The heads of units and services then submit their needs to the appropriate departments, for example, pay or the general management for needs exceeding a certain amount.With regard to the financial management of the CHUY, there is a manual of procedures developed in August 2006 that describes and sets out the management rules. This manual, which describes the financial management procedures, sets out the rules for managing the supply of goods and services, the rules for managing revenue, the rules for managing the treasury and the rules for budget management. In the management of the supply of goods and services, orders, receipt of orders and payments of trade debts are managed. Orders, for example, are placed on the basis of a needs sheet and are managed differently by the financial affairs division and by the general manager, depending on whether the amount is less than or greater than five (05) million. In other words, it is the director who orders expenditures in excess of five million.

3.1.7. Management analysis

The Yaoundé University Hospital Center is a Public Administrative Institution (EPA) that carries out public service activities. According to Braconnier (2007), an EPA is created either to meet a wide variety of objectives, or to fulfil a mission of general interest or to optimize the exercise of a mission by a public person, or to associate other persons more directly in the exercise of certain missions. Because of their traditional mission of sovereignty or social action, EPAs are in principle subject to public administrative law. However, the general statute of Cameroonian EPAs does not establish such a principle. It is the common law regime that applies to CHUY. This is sufficient proof that disputes which may involve or engage the responsibility of this institution fall within the domain and competence of the judicial judge[23].

As an EPA, the CHUY benefits from an administrative autonomy that allows it to freely organize its management mode and to choose its managerial techniques in order to achieve the objectives and missions assigned to it by the State. However, it is necessary to recall that MINSANTE and MINFI exercise a technical and financial supervision for the regularity of the acts of this institution.

3.2. Methodological approach

In this part of the methodology, the processes used for data collection are highlighted.

3.2.1. Type of study

Our study is qualitative in nature and its purpose is to highlight the impact of health legislation on the management of first category hospitals, in this case the University Hospital of Yaoundé. For more precision, our research will be of the "case study" type. The purpose of the "case study" is to describe a phenomenon in its reality, in interaction with the environment, and to account for the interplay of factors involved, as well as the complexity and richness of the situation being observed (Nkoum, 2005). The environment in question here is legal, with a large number of legislative and regulatory texts that must be applied in health facilities such as the one that is the subject of our research.

3.2.2 Research Methodology

After reviewing a large number of methodological documents, we chose the systemic method. The systemic method is the study of the regulation and equilibrium of systems. It values a global approach by giving priority to interactions with the environment (Nkoum, 2005: 65). In this case, the rule of law is general and impersonal. Health legislation must be applied in a general way in a health facility such as the CHUY in order to improve existing managerial practices. This improvement in managerial practices allows for better patient care and also improves the image of the facility. Thus, health legislation is the fatal weapon for improving relations with patients and the outside world. The systemic method will therefore allow us to provide support scientific and legal to the change of management methods and patient satisfaction in hospitals in general and in particular at the University Hospital of Yaoundé.

3.2.3 Study population and criteria for selecting informants

The population or "parent population" is the set of all individuals who possess specific characteristics related to the objectives of a survey (Mayer and Ouellet, 1991) cited by Nkoum (2005). Since our research is qualitative and applicable in a hospital environment, and given the different articulations of our theme, our target population is composed of the staff of the CHUY who are able to provide us with clear and honest information related to our theme.

To participate in this study, some inclusion and exclusion criteria were defined.

➢ Inclusion criteria

Our study included the leaders, administrative and managerial staff, and personnel present at the CHUY during the period of our investigation. We chose this population because on the one hand, the administrative executives of the CHUY are responsible for defining strategies, management styles and making major decisions concerning the center; the heads of department and unit for the implementation of these policies and decisions, the staff on whom many texts and administrative acts are applied and for whom the consequences, effects and repercussions of the provisions of the various health legislations can be pertinently analyzed.

➢ Exclusion Criteria

We excluded from this survey any person mentioned in the previous section who expressly wished not to participate in our study. In addition, we excluded from our study any person who was not a member of the CHUY and who did not request services offered by this hospital.

3.2.4. Target population

For Nkoum (2005: 114), a researcher who is called upon to conduct qualitative research is advised to use "exemplary samples. For the author, there is no mathematical formula for determining the size of an exemplary sample. For some specialists, he writes, "what seems important is the saturation point. Once the threshold is reached, it is almost useless to continue observing people or phenomena, because one risks repeating the same findings by observing the same thing. Nothing new will be collected once the saturation point is reached, he adds. In our study, we reached saturation after the twelfth ($12th$) interview because we realized that the interview responses were repetitions or repeated responses from previous interviews.

3.2.5. Study variables

Our study has two (02) variables: a dependent variable and an independent variable.

➢ **Dependent variable**

The effective and efficient management of the Yaoundé University Hospital is the dependent variable of our study.

➢ **Independent variables**

The independent variables of our research are health legislation, its enforcement, good governance practices[24] (Simo Kouam, 2015: 107).

3.2.6. Data collection instrument

The collection instrument refers to the medium, the intermediary that the researcher uses to collect the data to be submitted for analysis. The research instrument is a special technical package that the researcher will usually have to develop in order to meet specific research needs in terms of information whose processing will lead to the set objectives. The semi-structured interview makes it possible to collect specific information of various types f r o m one or more people, facts and verification of facts, information about the people involved, and information about the research. The interview guide used in this study allowed us to introduce our theme in the form of open-ended questions, leaving the respondent free to express himself and even to expand the subject. In this study, we used an interview guide that allowed us to introduce our theme in the form of open-ended questions, leaving the respondent free to express himself or herself and even to expand the subject. In addition, an observation grid of the functioning of the CHUY allowed us to better identify and understand what the surveys did not admit about certain aspects related to the management style and problems related to the application of health legislation. It should also be noted that documentary research was carried out outside and inside the study environment. It was necessary to analyze the impact of health legislation on the management of the CHUY, based on the legal texts identified. It also allowed us to review the works and publications already carried out on the theme.

3.2.5 The Observation Technique

According to Nkoum (2005), direct observation allows the researcher to collect data directly, without involving the subjects concerned by the survey. For this second data collection instrument, the observation grid, we chose non-participant observation because it allows the investigator to be more objective and to collect more objective data than participant observation (Nkoum, 2005).

3.2.6 Feasibility and validity test of the data collection device

➢ **Pre-test**

Researchers generally use pre-testing to ensure the reliability, feasibility of the study and the validity of the data in their studies. To this end, we submitted our interview guide to five (05) CHUY agents or personnel. These were excluded from the rest of the survey. Following this pre-test, some modifications were made and adopted.

➢ **Duration of the survey**

Our investigation which started on September 14, 2015 after an internship in Financial Analysis at CHUY ended on November 13, 2015. It therefore lasted 08 (eight) weeks and 04 (four) days.

3.2.7 Research ethics and scientific rigor

➢ Research ethics

For our study, obtaining research authorization from the Director of the SSE/UCAC and from the Deputy Director General of the CHUY is part of an ethical approach. During the data collection period, we sought informed consent from the informants so that we could receive fair information in return. The surveys were therefore free to withdraw from the study without having to justify themselves or provide explanations. We also ensured the confidentiality of the surveys.

➢ Scientific rigor

Thus, during our study, we first sought the consent of the investigators. Then, we explained the topic to them in a clear and fair way in order to obtain reliable and safe data. In doing so, we facilitated our easy acceptance. After the survey, we faithfully summarized the information obtained to each participant so that he/she could confirm, validate or invalidate it. The duration of the interview varied between 15 and 20 minutes depending on the availability of the interviewer and his or her level of understanding of our questions. However, some participants found it very interesting and enjoyable to discuss the topic with us, which justifies the long duration of some interviews[25].

3.2.8 Data collection method

> The interview

The interview was our main data collection technique. During our study, we submitted our interview guide to our interviewees on the theme of the impact of health legislation on the management of the Yaoundé University Hospital Center. They answered our questions freely. Without interrupting our interviewees, we only asked them the next question when we were satisfied with their answer. In this way, each question could lead to others. We recorded the data with a pen in the section of our interview guide reserved for this exercise. We also used our cell phone, which has a large capacity data recording system. At the end of each interview, a summary was given to the respondent for verification, modification or validation.

➢ The observation grid

To obtain information from our informants, we also used non-participant observation. By visiting different departments, we were able to observe the staff throughout the day and during their daily tasks. This technique allowed us to review the choice of our surveys, to better make this choice for a quality interview. The interview was conducted individually, intuitu personae, i.e., on a personal basis. Before starting the interview, the informants were given explanations on the theme, the purpose and the reason for the research and the interview. Reassured that our study could contribute to the improvement of the management of the CHUY and that the respect of the rights and freedoms of all parties could be observed, the informants were willing to participate in our exercise.

3.2.9 Analysis method: content analysis

With reference to the specific objectives of this qualitative research, we resorted to a content analysis. According to Morfaux (1980: 17-18), cited by Nkoum (2005), content analysis is "the objective, exhaustive, methodical and, if possible, quantitative examination of material, either verbal (information or texts: vocabulary, syntax, style, themes, etc.) or non-verbal (images, posters, gestures, mimicry, attitudes, voice), with a view to classifying and interpreting its elements. Since the data collected from the interviews and the observation grid were qualitative in nature, we grouped them and transformed them into items. We then proceeded to divide the elements of the informants' discourse into units of meaning and finally carried out an inventory and categorization according to the analysis model.

3.2.10 Difficulties encountered

The first difficulty is related to the geographical accessibility of the CHUY. Indeed, we live in Soa. During our research, it was necessary for us to be at the CHUY before the time scheduled for the beginning of the work, in order to observe certain practices that the surveys could not identify. Another difficulty is the difficult access to information. Moreover, interpersonal communication is a major problem in this health facility. In addition to this problem, there is the problem of the availability of management tools from the CHUY. The documentation was not accessible and some people did not fail to tell us that the documents of the CHUY could not be within our reach. Some officials of this Hospital and University Center also told us that the documents of this center cannot be in the hands of a student. Finally, our financial situation was a major difficulty in the success of this study.

3.2.11 Limitations of the study

The human work is not perfect. Our research inevitably has some limitations. First, our acceptance at UHC was not easy. Some informants even had to send us away after agreeing to the study, thinking that we were investigating on behalf of the director general.[26] At the time of our investigation, some informants were not yet in the office. At the time of our survey, some informants were not available, which led us to change them. This prevented us from obtaining some important data for our research.

3.2.12 Counting and presentation of results

The counting of the results was done manually at the end of our survey. For this purpose, materials such as pens, pencils, formats, rulers, were used. These data were presented in synthetic tables that we will present in the next chapter.

➢ Data analysis

Qualitative data analysis is more subjective than quantitative analysis (Nkoum, 2005). Saturation and validation aim to objectify the first analysis. In our study, we used saturation to analyze our data. According to the above-mentioned author, saturation indicates that the desired level has been reached. The researcher can then end his or her collection, assuming that he or she has seen what there is to see. It is said that "saturation is reached when the investigation of reality no longer brings anything new" (Nkoum, 2005). During our investigation, the surveys used a routine vocabulary referring to the same reality, which allows us to conclude that the saturation threshold has been reached.

3.2.13 Communication of results

Nkoum (2005) wrote "for a research work to take on a scientific status, it is fundamental that its results be published, i.e., submitted to the criticism of the scientific community". After having given a copy to the coordinators of the work, the communication of the results of this study is done in the following way
- Handing in the copy to the members of the jury;

- The presentation of the results in front of a jury as part of the defense of our thesis;
- Handing in the copy to the ESS/UCAC library after correction;

- Handing in the copy to the management of the CHUY after correction

CHAPTER 4
PRESENTATION OF RESULTS

In this chapter, we will faithfully present the data we collected in the field from the survey that was conducted from September 14 to November 13, 2015. These data were recorded using a cell phone, pen and paper. We then transcribed the recordings and grouped them according to the objectives of the study. Our analysis is descriptive, meaning it is based on content analysis. In other words, it is about highlighting the different concepts from the research and analyzing them in more depth.

4.1 Presentation of the results of the interview guide

These results include the following:

4.1.1 Survey profile;

Table 6: Presentation of surveys by gender

Type	Workforce
Female	04
Male	08
Total	12

The male gender predominates in our target population. Out of twelve (12) surveys, we had eight (08) men and four (04) women.

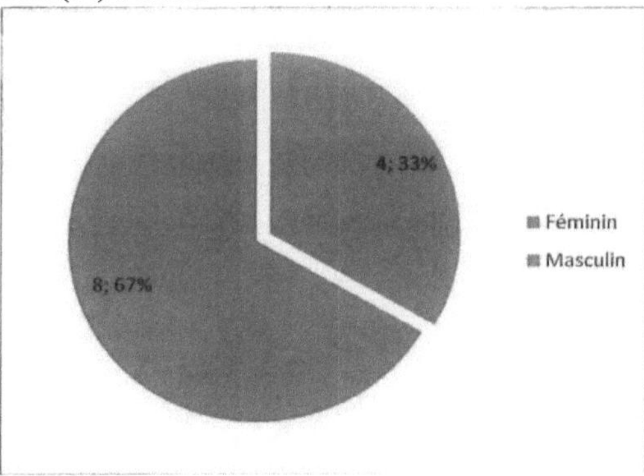

Figure 2: Graphical presentation of respondents by gender

Table 7: Representation of surveys by education level

Level of instruction	Workforce
Primary	01
Secondary	01
Superior	10
Total	12

The majority of our surveys are made up of higher education graduates: 10 out of 12 informants. The secondary level is not much represented, i.e. 01 out of 12 informants, as well as the primary level represented by only one (01) person.

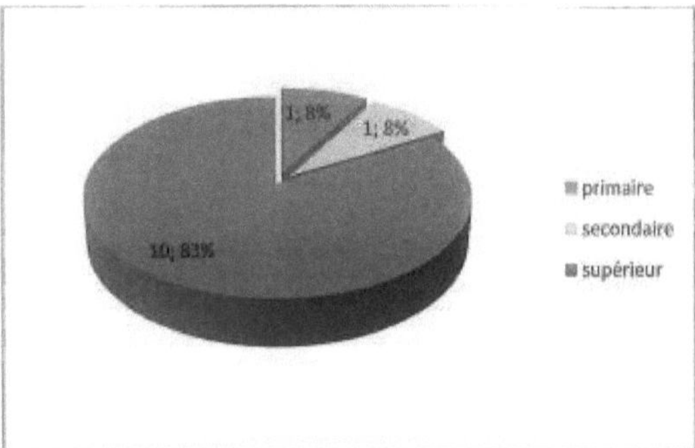

Figures 3: Graphical representation of respondents by level of education

Table 8: Presentation of surveys by function

Function/qualification professional	Workforce
Administrative	06
Nursing staff	03
Support staff	03
Total	12

The table shows us that 06 people are administrative managers, heads of division and services and assimilated, 03 nursing staff and 03 support staff.

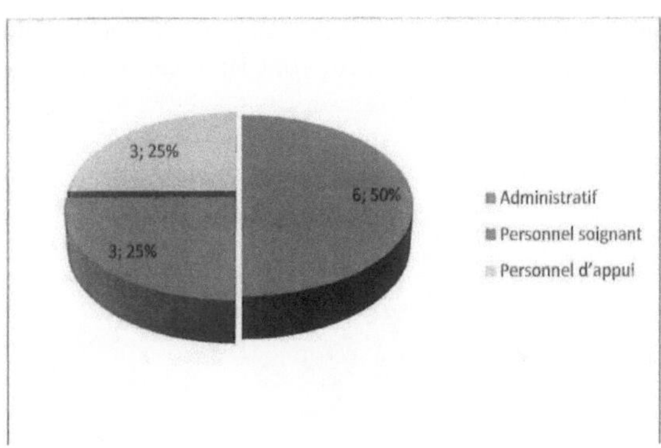

Figure 4: Graphical representation of respondents by function

Table 9: Presentation of surveys by nature of commitment

Nature of commitment	Workforce
Public servant	04
Contractual	08
Total	12

We can observe the predominance of contract workers in our target population. That is to say 08 Contractuals against 04 civil servants for a sample of 12 informants.

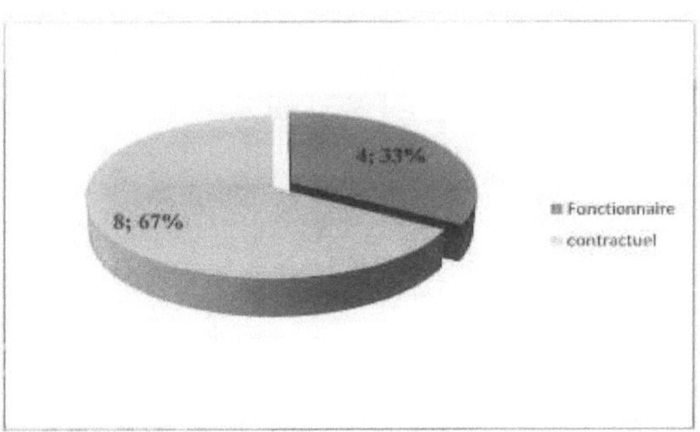

Figure 5: Graphical representation of respondents according to the nature of the commitment

Table 10: Presentation of surveys by seniority

Seniority	Workforce
Less than 10 years old	04
From 10 to 20 years	04
From 20 to 30 years old	02
Over 30 years old	02
Total	12

In our parent population, 08 surveys are older than 10 years. We are therefore confident that the individuals surveyed have a good knowledge of CHUY and can provide us with reliable information on our topic.

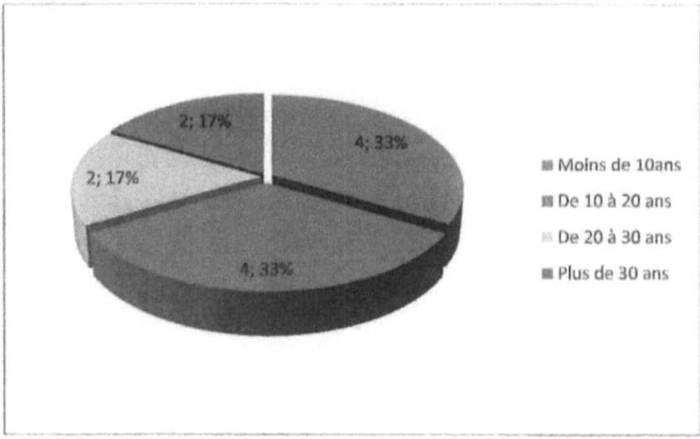

Figure 6: Graphical representation of respondents according to seniority

Table 11: Survey presentation by region of origin

Region of origin	Workforce
North	01
South	02
Center	04
East	01
West	02
Coastal	01
Southwest	01
Total	12

In our sample, nationals from the Central region are in the majority with a total of 04 informants, followed by the Western and Southern regions with 02 surveys each, and the Coastal, Northern, Eastern and Southwestern regions with 01.

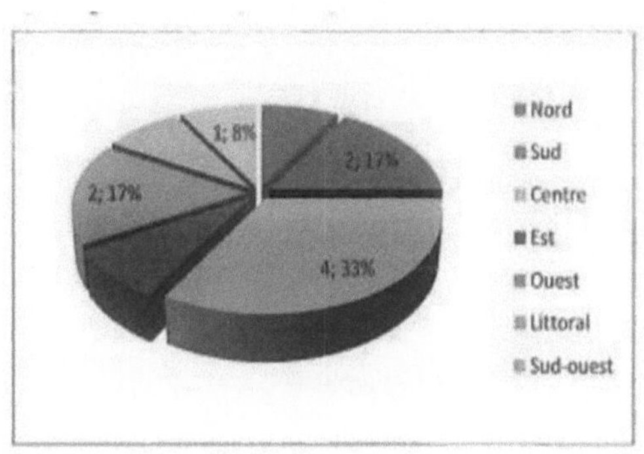

Figure 7: Graphical representation of respondents by region of origin

Table 12: Survey presentation by ethnicity

Ethnicity	Workforce
Eton	02
Bonkcng	01
Fong	01
Bamileké	01
Bamoum	01
Bassa	01
Bayangui	01
Boulou	01
Éwondo	01
Kako	01
Mound Ang	01
Total	12

There is an equitable representation of the ethnic groups in our population with a slight predominance of the Etons (02 surveys).

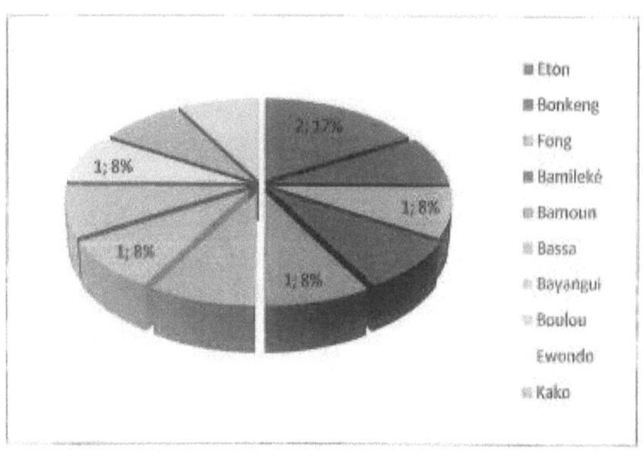

Figure 8: Representation of respondents by ethnicity

4.1.2 The current state of health legislation applicable in first category hospitals (case of the CHUY)

Table 13: Legal texts applicable to CHUY

	Information
	"The texts applicable to UHC are numerous. They are generally laws, statutes, establishment contracts, etc."
	"There are a lot of texts that apply to UHC."
	"I do not have sufficient knowledge of the texts applicable to the UHC.
	"I have a partial knowledge of the texts applicable to the CHUY. But I know that the general statute of the civil service applies to civil servants.and contractual workers the labour code "
	"At CHUY, we apply laws such as the finance law, many decrees like those on the reorganization of CHUY, the general status of EPA, the status of the public sector, the labor code and many others. others "
	"There is a plurality of texts that UHC should apply. Doing the It is not easy for me to identify these texts.
	"There are many texts that in principle should apply to UHC, to which are added the decisions taken internally".
	"At CHUY we have the texts of the state in their entirety such as
	laws, decrees, circulars and instructions, statutes. We also have the establishment agreements, the statute of the CHUY, the lower regulations, the resolutions of the board of directors, all the decisions,circulars, memos, etc..
	"The texts are numerous; those that apply to the UHC are even more numerous because, apart from those that we know, others are created by the masters of the house who impose them on the least of these we "

	"At UHC we have texts of general scope and texts of specific scope. The texts of general scope are the laws and decrees that can be applied at the same time to the CHUY and to all other non hospital: the finance law, the general status of the EPAs. The texts of
	The specific scope of these regulations applies only to the UHC: the decree on the organization and operation of the UHC "
	"Time will not permit us to cite all the texts that apply to the CHUY. Nevertheless, the laws such as the finance laws, the framework law on health, the decrees, the orders of the ministries of health, of higher education, of finance, and even of commerce, to name but a few, apply to CHUY. In addition to these texts, the decisions of the board of directors, those of the director as well as all the other acts are applicable administrative measures taken by CHUY officials".
	"I do not have a perfect knowledge of the health legislation that applies to the UHC, but I know that civil servants and contractuals are treated differently, which means that the texts that the texts are different "

Clearly, there are several types of legal texts applicable to UHC. This is what the vast majority of the surveys made us understand. For some, "There is a plurality of texts that the CHUY should apply. It is not easy for me to identify these texts," said the sixth informant in our study. These texts can be of general or specific scope: "At the UHC we have texts of general scope and texts of specific scope. The texts of general scope are the laws and decrees that can be applied at the same time to the CHUY and to all other non-hospital establishments: the finance law, the general status of the EPAs. The texts of specific scope do not apply only to the CHUY: the decree on the organization and functioning of the CHU" explained another respondent.

Table 14: Timeliness, adaptability and volume of texts

-	Information
	"The texts are numerous but for the most part, poorly adapted"
	"The texts must be adapted and updated to better serve the management of CHUY"
	"I don't think that texts should be adapted to UHC, it is the latter that should adapt to the texts.
	"I think it would be better for the nursing staff to have a special regime. This will allow the legislator to make laws adapted to the hospital sector which until now has been neglected and left in the hands of outlawed "
	"The texts applied by CHUY are circumstantial texts that do not do not suffer from a problem of updating. On the other hand, it would be preferable to adapt these texts to our hospital which is an EPA like no other.
	"The problem is not the volume of legislation applicable to UHC, much less the timeliness of the texts, the problem is the application of these texts "
	"The texts are sufficient. But we would benefit from updating them and adapting them to UHC."
	"There are very good texts in Cameroon, the problem is the human resources responsible for applying them.
	"The volume of texts is sufficient, they just need to be updated and adapted to UHC."
	"A significant number of texts applicable in primary care hospitals are category in Cameroon, like the CHUY, are neither updated nor adapted to their management".
	"First class hospitals such as UHC fundamentally deserve a better framework.
	"You can't adapt texts to each particular situation, that would be a double standard. Perhaps they need to be updated.

The number of legal texts applicable to UHC is significant but requires adaptation. This is what emerges from the testimonies of the surveys. For example, for one respondent, "The texts are sufficient. But we would benefit from updating them and adapting them to UHC. According to some other informants, these texts also deserve to be updated: "The texts must be adapted and updated in order to better serve the management of CHUY," suggested one informant. For another respondent, it is just a problem of applying the texts. Yet another respondent supports the idea of the need for a better legal framework for first category hospitals such as CHUY.

Table 15: The capacity of health legislation to boost the managerial efficiency of CHUY

	Information
	"The texts are taken in a state of law like ours to allow the proper functioning of institutions. A good application of these texts can inevitably boost the managerial effectiveness of UHC."
	"All legislation is intended to improve either the organization or the functioning of a society. Health legislation can boost efficiency management of the CHUY "
	"Texts alone cannot build or develop, let alone make the care. The will to develop comes from Man and not from the texts "
	"Health legislation is enacted to be enforced in order to improve the results of a sector. The one applicable to CHUY has this capacity to boost efficiency management of the center "
	"Once adapted and properly applied, the texts will make a considerable contribution to the growth of CHUY"
	"Health legislation can boost the managerial effectiveness of UHC if and only if it is well applied".
	"The existing legal texts can boost the managerial efficiency of the CHUY. But it is necessary to update and adapt them.
	"The strict and firm application of the texts and the judicious choice of resources human resources can boost the managerial effectiveness of UHC.
	"The arsenal of existing legal standards can turn UHC into a hospital paradise if the men respect the texts "
	"On the one hand, health legislation can enable better management of the CHUY when it is perfectly applied. On the other hand, the texts themselves
	The same factors are a hindrance to the managerial efficiency of UHC.
	"Enable UHC to boost its managerial efficiency, increase its and to achieve its objectives, this is the main role of the legislation".
	"Boosting the managerial efficiency of the CHUY is a matter for the leaders of this hospital institution. The texts can only frame their efforts.

Undoubtedly, the legal texts applicable to CHUY can boost the managerial efficiency of this hospital formation. This assertion stems from the information gathered from the survey crowd. Some of them also set a condition for these texts to boost the managerial efficiency of CHUY. Thus, they need to be adapted and updated: "Once they are adapted and properly applied, the texts will make a considerable contribution to the growth of CHUY," as one respondent put it. For other informants, the texts alone cannot allow CHUY to develop; they must be combined with "a human will". However, one of our informants believes that legislation can both enable the development of CHUY and hinder it: "On the one hand, health legislation can enable better management of CHUY when it is perfectly applied. On the other hand, the texts themselves are a hindrance to the managerial efficiency of CHUY.

Table 16: What can be done to ensure that health legislation allows for the development of CHUY

	Information
	"We must first disclose the health legislation and then apply it normally and look for gaps".
	"Those who have to apply it should be equipped and it should be better explained to others because some people make mistakes because they know it. badly or not at all "
	"Training, awareness of the legislation and compliance with it can ensure that the texts allow UHC to develop."
	"People have to respect the texts and the decisions made by the top hierarchy."
	"The proper application of appropriate legislation will allow the development of UHC.
	"The texts are made to be applied and only the application of these can change things"
	"Existing health care legislation can of course enable the development of UHC if it is implemented."
	"We must ensure the rigorous application of the texts and a judicious choice of human resources".
	"The establishment of an efficient and effective governing body, with people who have a knowledge of law and management, to ensure that this is done. the application of the legislation at UHC".
	"It is necessary to adapt and update and then apply the texts in an environment hospital environment marked by the urgency of immediate care".
	"Existing legislation can allow UHC to grow if it is properly implemented."
	"Texts must be taken with the aim of orienting human action".

In spite of the adaptation and updating of health legislation to allow for the development of CHUY, the surveys believe that it should be well implemented. For some of these informants, it is also important to make a judicious choice of human resources with the capacity to promote the development of CHUY.

4.1.3 The application of health legislation

Table 17: Assessment of the application of health legislation at UHC

Information
"So far, the health legislation is partially applied at the CHUY. This is due to the ignorance of the texts".
"It is very badly applied. We don't have the impression that we have the texts in this hospital. Some decisions are made with the aim of harming "
"The application of the legislation at UHC is average. It's mostly because of this that people do not know the texts".
"The legislation is not respected at all at the CHUY. It is even sometimes applied to the headhunter and depends on your relationship with the boss."
"Misapplication of the legislation insofar as it is not fair. Maybe because they don't know the texts.
"If UHC is not doing well, it is because everyone is doing what they want. The legislation is more than ever poorly enforced".
"Legislation is autocratically enforced at UHC. The leaders have created legislation that suits them".
"The application of health legislation at the CHUY is null. It is the non respect of the legislation that prevails at the CHUY. It is mainly bad faith that justifies this bad application of the texts.
"The application of the legislation is not at all good at UHC, I would even say it is fragmented, personal, not impartial."
"The application of health legislation is controversial at UHC. The The poor application of the sanitary legislation is explained by the ignorance of the texts which translates the incompetence of our leaders".
"The application of existing texts at UHC is poor. Management does not do not know the legislation that must be applied to UHC."
"I don't even know if we apply the texts at CHUY".

Clearly, the application of health legislation is poor, non-existent, partial or even controversial at UHC. This is what emerges from the information collected from 9 out of 12 surveys. However, 2 surveys found this application to be partial. This poor application can be justified firstly by ignorance of the texts: "The application of The existing texts at the CIIUY are poor. The leaders do not know the legislation that must apply to the CHUY" he told us another investigation. It is then justified, according to our informants, by bad faith. It is in this respect that an interviewee declared strongly that : "The application of health legislation at the CHUY is null. It is the non-respect of the legislation that prevails at CHUY. It is especially the bad faith which justifies this bad application of the texts ".

Table 18: Achievement of results with regard to the application of health legislation at UHC

	Information
	"When the standard is flouted, the results will only be poor. UHC cannot achieve results in a mess, in l Injustice."
	"At CHUY, the staff is not motivated, therefore the results cannot be achieved.
	"The legislation is poorly applied. Results are tainted, mediocrity wins over results, work is burdensome and not a duty".
	"The legislation (as it is applied) cannot allow UHC to achieve the results."
	"No institution can achieve its results in the absence of well-constructed legislation"
	"Poor enforcement at UHYC can't produce good results."
	"Results hardly achieved with regard to the application of the legislation".
	"The application of health legislation at UHC may push the staff to go beyond the results".
	"Results will be achieved if legislation is enforced"
	"The general texts do not always allow for the achievement of the expected results at UHC. However, the results cannot be This is the only way to ensure the safety of the people in this facility because the legislation is not being enforced.
	"If legislation is going to enable UHC to achieve its goals, then it should be enforced."
	"With or without text, it is difficult for UHC to achieve its results because of the performance of the leadership team."

Undoubtedly, the application of health legislation cannot allow UHC to achieve its results. The majority of informants agreed to relax this view. Thus, according to one of these surveys. "The legislation as it is applied cannot allow CHUY to achieve the results."

Table 19: What needs to be done to improve health enforcement practices at UHC

	Information
	"We should match the position with the profile of the applicants (lawyers in their place, doctors in their positions), redeploy the staff according to the skills"
	"First of all, this legislation must be well organized, and then the staff must be trained and informed on the subject.
	"Equip themselves with legislative and legal knowledge, train staff and implement a compliant action plan with indicators
	"Health legislation should be restructured, reorganized and adapted to the hospital environment; competent people should be chosen for its application"
	"We need to strengthen the legal and regulatory framework and train staff."
	"Uniformity and promotion of the texts, i.e. sensitization of the personnel".
	"Consolidate the texts, update them, adapt them, make them known, change leadership, appointing appropriate administrators, etc.."
	"The real involvement of the state, that the state puts everything back to normal and that the choice of human resources be judicious at UHC.
	"We need to harmonize the texts. We also need all staff to applies the legislation "
	"It is necessary first to restructure and reorient the hospital sub-sector, then to harmonize the legal system adapted to this sector to finally ensure its application by men of justice and integrity".
	"We must accustom the staff to the use and application of the texts in force"
	"Staff must do what is expected of them, they must meet the standards prescribed by the state."

Restructuring or better framing of health legislation seems to be the common wish of our surveys: **"First of all**, the hospital sub-sector must be restructured and reoriented, then the legal system adapted to this sector must be harmonized, and finally its application must be ensured by people of justice and integrity. These words express the desire of an informant to see a better framework, a better legal organization of the health sector and the hospital sub-sector. Also, the rigorous choice of the men who should apply this legislation well is added to this wish: "To gather the texts, to update them, to adapt them, to make them known, to change leadership, to appoint competent administrators, etc.", adds another.

4.1.4 The effects of health legislation on the management of CHUY

Table 20: The management style of CHUY

	Information
	"The management style is directive at CHUY. Senior management makes all the decisions. But UHC is large and this style is not appropriate. not"
	"When the director is there, he makes all the decisions, but when he is absent, some people do as they please".
	"It's an authoritarian management. Staff are not always involved in making certain decisions that affect them.
	"management is anarchic at CHUY"
	An archaic management, a "messy" management: that's what we can say about the management of the CHUY".
	"I often wonder if we have texts in this hospital. Nothing is structured or organized at CHUY, the Director and his team do whatever they want. want and we suffer".
	"Management at CHUY is autocratic. The chief decides on everything and the subordinates suffer.
	"Authoritarian style characterizes management at CHUY"
	"It's fuzzy management"
	"Management at CHUY is directive and mostly vertical. A style that does not does not fit with the size of the CHUY".
	"Management is an authoritarian style at UHC. Decisions are made at the top and implemented with or without possible explanation."
	"At CHUY, it's a dictatorship

The lexical field used by the majority of our informants on the management style refers to the directive style of management. Some of them clearly stated it in our interview: "The management style is directive at the CHUY. The general management makes all the decisions. However, UHC is large and this style is not appropriate," one interviewee stated forcefully. Others use rather harsh terms to characterize this management: "The authoritarian style characterizes the management of the CHUY," confided another informant. For still others, the management style applied by CHUY is not understood by the staff: "It is a vague management" according to an informed respondent. According to another informant, the management applied at CHUY is comparable to a dictatorship: "At CHUY, it's a dictatorship," he said.

Table 21: The characteristic of the management of CHUY

	Information
	"CHUY management is characterized by disorder, failure, and descent into hell."
	"It's a bad management, I would even say a catastrophic management.
	"Whoever does not involve his employees in the management of his establishment is doomed to failure. That's what happened to our beautiful hospital.
	"CHUY management is anarchic and does not respect any standards"
	"The disorder is the main characteristic of the management of the CHUY. It is dominated by the non-respect of the texts in force in our country".
	"it's a catastrophic management".
	"Management at CHUY is autocratic. The chief decides on everything and the subordinates suffer.
	"It's a bad management, a chaotic management similar to the management of the neighborhood grocery store.
	"Unclear management is management that no one can understand. This is the type of management that applies to UHC.
	"it is a management of '7 'opacity' (see A TEBA EYENE Charles) ".
	"UHC management is totalitarian, a management of chaos."
	"It's dictatorship instead of management"

By collecting data from our surveys, we obviously understand that the management of the CHUY is chaotic, catastrophic, characterized by disorder, vagueness and the cult of failure. Although some informants did not express this clearly, one of them did not hesitate to specify that "It is bad management, chaotic management similar to the management of the neighborhood grocery store.

Table 22: The impact of the application of the legislation on the management of CHUY

	Information
	"mediocrity, disorder, chaos are the effects of such an application of the texts".
	"the consequences are: discontent, uprisings, bad work"
	"The repercussions are numerous: the lack of a shared objective, repeated mistakes, sanctions, poor performance, and the loss of a job. uprisings "
	"In this situation, the repercussions will only be negative: the staff has a lot of pressure, a permanent fear of being sanction; etc.."
	"The salary arrears and quotas, the precariousness of the personnel, the dysfunction of the institution".
	"chaos, nothing works at CHUY"
	"The demotivation of the staff, the lack of stock of inputs. quality of delivery and service "
	"It's chaos, strikes, demotivation, poor delivery (UHC is minus infinity)"
	"unpaid salaries and quotas, human rights violated
	"it's the poor functioning of the hospital, poor care patients, lack of better student mentoring and continuing education for staff.
	"The effects are negative, it is the sinking of the CLIUY
	"everyone complains, staff situation to be desired"

When legislation is poorly applied, its effects are very negative in the management of a hospital structure such as CHUY. One informant summarized these effects in the following terms: "the hospital does not function well, patients are not treated well, there is no better supervision of students and no better continuous training of staff".

Table 23: The impact of health legislation on the management of CHUY

	Information
	"Health legislation in itself can have a positive influence on the management of CHUY, but its application within this training hospital management is negatively impacted".
	"legislation is intended to regulate an industry, but its application at the CHUY has as consequences: discontent, uprisings, poor performance".
	"the health legislation as it is applied has negatively impacted the management of the CHUY all these last years "
	"Poorly implemented legislation will only have a negative impact on management.
	"the application of health legislation at the CHUY cannot give expected results and therefore negatively impact the management".
	"Legislation is taken to positively influence the management of the CHUY, but when it is badly applied, as is the case, management is catastrophic.
	"The legislation as applied to UHC has not been effective.
	"Health legislation should allow for the development of CHUY. Such as that it is applied, it has a negative impact on UHC in that it leads to more chaos.
	"as applied, health legislation is having a negative impact at UHC"
	"Generally, legislation is intended to organize and regulate a sector of activity. In this case, it has a positive impact on the management of the structure. However, its application at the CHUY produces negative effects in this hospital facility".
	"poor enforcement of legislation is hurting UHC".
	"the impact of health legislation is not good at UHC".

Our informants recognize the purpose of health legislation to organize, regulate and allow the development of an activity or a sector, but the legislation applicable to the CHUY can in no way positively impact the management of this health and university training. More than 7 surveys unanimously share this position.

4.2. Presentation of the results of the observation grid

We used non-participant observation for our grid because of our lack of qualification in health care. However, the administration of the CHUY authorized our visit to the services to observe certain practices at the same time as we were able to pass our interview guide. Our observation grid therefore focused on certain practices related to compliance with health legislation at the UHC. Thus, we propose this observation grid.

Table 24: Observation grid

The Indicators	The standard	The practice	The gap/observation
Time of arrival at work	07h 30min	Between 08h and 09h	Varies between 30min and 01 h 30min delay, schedules not respected
Start time of work	08h	08h 30min-09h 30min	30min-01h 30min late, no schedule respected
Time of Processing of files that do not have a financial impact	24 to 48 hours	More than 48 hours	Deadlines not met
Time of Treatment of Files having a financial impact	72 hours	More than 72 hours	Deadlines not met
Working time	08 h-09 h of work in day	Less time at the work	Some useless ballads in the corridors
Communication interpersonal	Posting notes on the bulletin board	Few people stop to get information	Lack of information
Communication with patients	Delivery of clear information and loyal	Verbal aggression, frustration,	Disregard for patient's rights
Remuneration and motivation of the staff	Staff are entitled to remuneration and certain benefits such as quotas. shares	Complaints from more than 5 staff in our presence during the training period and data collection	Workers' rights not respected
Type	Gender Equality	Predominance of male sex	Discrimination on the basis of female gender
Alternation	Status of EPAs: the mandate of the CEO is for (Bans renewable) 02 times	From 1999 to 2015	
Allocation of quotas	Distribution of shares according to responsibility, on-call and		
	attendance, punctuality, helpfulness and probity;		

CHAPTER 5
SYNTHESIS AND DISCUSSION

This chapter aims to make sense of the results presented above. It also aims to confront these results with the theories that have been invoked. Therefore, it is appropriate to highlight the synthesis and discussion of the results of our study according to the themes and sub-themes in line with our objectives.

5.1 Survey Profile 5.1.1 Gender

Gender is an important motive to consider in our survey. It defends Today, gender equality is a principle that is recognized at both the international and national levels. At the international level, the Charter of the United Nations of 1945 displays in its preamble a completely innovative profession of faith: "We the peoples of the United Nations determined to (...) reaffirm faith in fundamental human rights, in the dignity and worth of the human person, in the equal rights of men and women and of nations large and small. The Universal Declaration of Human Rights of 1948 seems to follow in the footsteps of its article 21 paragraph 2 which states that "everyone has the right of equal access to public service in his country". At the national level, the Constitution of June 2, 1972, revised by Law No. 96/06 of January 18, 1996, itself amended and completed by Law No. 2008/001 of April 14, 2008, unambiguously enshrines the principle of equality between all men without distinction of any kind, particularly on the basis of gender, in the following terms: "all men (men and women) are equal in rights and duties" and "each person must participate in proportion to his or her abilities in public office.[27]. In our survey, we have more men than women. This can obviously reflect an imbalance or discrimination based on gender in recruitment. At UHC, the predominance of males over females does not seem to pose any problem. problem to the administrators of this center. During our visit to the various departments in this health facility, we regretfully made our observation on the predominance of men at the CHUY known to certain senior managers. Against all odds, they told us that we would be better off "dealing with the real problems than wasting time comparing the number of men to the number of women working at themCHUY. Notwithstanding, it would therefore be important for CHUY leaders to develop policies to take gender into account in the various recruitment processes.

5.1.2 Education level and function

In an organization chart, the function defines the permanent objectives, the main tasks, the competencies, the means used and the hierarchical and operational relationships linked to the achievement of results by the organization's personnel. The levels of qualification allow for positioning in relation to the job market and the ability to achieve the expected results. Thus, the holder of a qualification is assumed to be able to occupy a position requiring the knowledge and skills corresponding to a diploma. This means, therefore, that the level of education allows for the acquisition of a certain competence that gives rise to the granting of a given function. In this perspective, the notion of competence deserves to be understood. Competence refers to the mobilization of a set of resources, including knowledge, know-how and interpersonal skills, in order to resolve a complex situation (Roegiers, 2010). For Levy-Leboyer (2009), competence is "the integrated implementation of skills, personality traits and

53

also acquired knowledge, in order to carry out a complex mission within the framework of the company that has entrusted the individual with it, and in the spirit of its strategies and culture. The level of education is therefore a promoter of competence for access to a position. Apart from the results of the profile presented above, our observation shows that at the CHUY, there is not a perfect match between the level of education and the position held. In the theory of the administrative function, Fayol insisted on the need for those in charge of an organization to acquire administrative or even management training in order to better fulfill their functions or perform their tasks. It would then be more profitable for this university hospital institution to redistribute positions according to the qualifications of the personnel and especially to set up a real policy of continuous training.

5.1.3 The nature of the commitment

The nature of the employment allows us to classify the personnel in an organization. In our study, almost all of the personnel surveyed at CHUY were recruited on the basis of an employment contract governed by common law, more precisely labor law. Since civil servants are not very well represented, we tend to say that common law texts are applied in the majority of cases at CHUY. This consideration is not simply a remark by the researcher. Article 10 paragraph 1 (b) of the General Statute of the Civil Service excludes the application of the said statute to agents of parapublic organizations and public establishments of an administrative nature. As a reminder, the CHUY is a public administrative establishment. However, the predominance of contract staff and the exclusion of the application of the general statute of the Cameroonian civil service can have serious consequences on the management of the finances of the center. The more important the personnel file is, the more serious the expenses become. This can create an imbalance between available resources and staff expectations. It should be remembered that the hospital center has, in recent years, been characterized by numerous staff demands, often leading to uprisings and announcements or the launching of strikes.

5.1.4 Seniority

The majority of informants in our sample had more than 10 years of work experience at UHC. Seniority in a department can be an asset to the management of the department in the sense that staff acquire, over time, technical skill, mastery of certain files and increased professional experience. However, when we talk about seniority or the number of years of high service in a department or in the administration of an organization, the problem of alternation arises in the minds of some critics. For these critics, it is necessary to alternate in order to give others the opportunity to apply their skills (knowledge, know-how, interpersonal skills). However, alternation does not seem to be the most common practice at CHUY. Indeed, law n°99/016 of 22 December 19991 on the General Statute of Public Establishments and Enterprises in the public and parapublic sector stipulates in its article 68 that "the Director General (of an EPA) is appointed by decree of the President of the Republic for a period of three (3) years, renewable two (2) times". An observation from our grid shows that the Director General has been appointed to head this EPA since 1999 and was only relieved of this function during our data collection period.

5.1.5 The region and the ethnicity

In Cameroon, the policy of regional balance is formalized jointly by Decree No. 82/407 of September 7, 1982, which gave carte blanche to the Minister of Public Service to define the quotas and Order No. 10467 signed by the Minister of Public Service on

October 4, 1982, updated on August 20, 1992. Article 2 of this decree, reproduced in Article 60 of Decree No. 2000/696/PM of September 13, 2000 establishing the system of administrative competitions, provides for 5% of places in Adamaoua, 18% in the far north, 7% in the north, 15% in the center, 4% in the east, 4% in the south, 13% in the west, 12% in the Littoral, 12% in the northwest and 8% in the southwest

This policy is cited in our study in order to highlight the representativeness of the provinces, now regions, in the management and operation of the CHUY. We want to make sure that the management of the CHUY is not reserved for one region, let alone one ethnic group. However, several regions seem to be represented but not in accordance with the regional balance.

5.2   The state of health legislation applicable in first category hospitals (case of CHUY)

Taking stock of the health legislation applicable to UHC Y seemed to be an exercise of some complexity for some of our investigations. In this study, knowledge of legal texts is not perfect at CHUY. Indeed, some felt that they did not have sufficient knowledge of the texts. Others acknowledged that they had an approximate or even average knowledge of the legal texts applicable in first category hospitals. Thus, "I don't have sufficient knowledge of the texts applicable to the UHC" confided to us an investigator. Another, limited himself to the following statement without making any effort to quote them: "There are many texts that apply to the UHC". These statements may, to some extent, lead us to believe that staff do not have a good knowledge of the legal texts applicable to CHUY. Moreover, our observation grid indicates that a limited number of personnel stop in front of the bulletin board to read the notes posted by the hospital administration. However, "no one is supposed to be ignorant of the law", the Cameroonian Penal Code recommends on the first cover. As such, these positions are out of phase with the pure theory of law which proposes a specific method of knowledge of the law. In the same vein, some informants have an advanced knowledge of the legislation applicable in first category hospitals, especially those considered as EPAs. In this respect, several of the interviewees seem to have mastered the texts in force. For the latter, these texts may be of general or specific scope:"At the CHUY we have texts of general scope and texts of specific scope. The texts of general scope are the laws and decrees that can be applied at the same time to the CHUY and to all other non-hospital establishments: the finance law, the general status of the EPA. Texts of specific scope apply only to CHUY: the decree on the organization and functioning of CHUY," explained a documented respondent. This can then allow us to classify and even rank these texts in accordance with the hierarchy of legal norms initiated by Kelsen.With respect to the volume, timeliness and adaptability of the legal texts applicable to CHUY, there seems to be a consensus among staff that the health legislation in our country should be reviewed. For most of the surveys, the number of legal texts applicable to CHUY is important but requires adaptation. Thus, one of these surveys suggested that, "the texts are sufficient. But we would benefit from updating them and adapting them to UHC. Similarly, for other informants, these texts also deserve to be updated: "The texts must be adapted and updated in order to better serve the management of CHUY," one informant suggested. The desire of informants to adapt, update, or even organize or codify texts that apply to first category hospitals obeys the legal positivism that wants there to be a physical, legal support for the standards that must be applied to a sector or field of activity. This codification is not the work of UHC, but rather of the legislator or public authorities. One of the contributions of this study will therefore be to propose a refoundation of the Cameroonian health system that will include a serious hospital reform of our legal framework. This reform of the Cameroonian health and hospital system must be based on relevant and necessary legal foundations for a better consideration and managerial practice. This idea can find its legal foundation in the legal positivism developed in the Pure Theory of Law of Kelsen. In the case of our study, can health legislation, although sufficient, be adapted, updated or even better framed to boost the managerial efficiency of an EPA hospital such as the CHUY? On the question of the capacity of health legislation to boost the managerial efficiency of CHUY, we received a conditional affirmation from our informants. Firstly, the legal texts applicable to the CHUY can boost the managerial efficiency of this hospital. This is what emerges from the information gathered from 5 out of 12 people surveyed at CHUY. Secondly, some surveys set a condition for these texts to boost the managerial efficiency of CHUY. Thus, they need to be adapted, updated and, above all, properly applied: "Once they are adapted and properly applied, the texts will make a considerable contribution to the growth of CHUY," is the prescription of one of the respondents. The need to apply the laws in order to boost the efficiency of CHUY is undoubtedly the wish of the informants, who believe that the laws alone are not enough; they must be combined with "a human will". Such a will is expressly expressed by another informant for whom "the strict and firm application of texts and the judicious choice of human resources can boost the managerial efficiency of the CHUY". This position is supported by Fayol's theory of the Administrative Function, which states that functions should be occupied by those who are competent to assume them. Finally, an interviewee believes that the texts can both allow the development of CHUY and hinder it: "On the one hand, health legislation can allow for better management of CHUY when it is perfectly applied. On the other hand, the texts themselves are a hindrance to the managerial efficiency of CHUY. According to the logic of our informant, the procedures relating to the awarding of contracts, for example, can have a negative influence on the management of a public hospital of the EPA rank insofar as the hospital is called upon to manage emergency cases which also require an emergency response. When a bulb burns out in an operating theatre, while the surgeon is in the middle of an operation, the procedures, however long they may be, can lead to the loss of one or more human lives. In the end, everything seems to depend on the application of the existing texts. This is what is strongly recommended by the pure theory of law in legal positivism, which ensures that norms are not only codified but also applied. In response, our surveys agreed to propose an approach to be followed so that the health legislation can allow the development of the CHUY. Thus, the majority of the surveys think that existing health legislation should first be properly applied. For other informants, it is also important to make a judicious choice of human resources with the capacity to promote the development of CHUY, such as as recommended by Fayol in his theory of the Administrative Function developed in the classical school of thought. Clearly, the inventory of health legislation applicable to first category hospitals reveals in our study of the CHUY that there are a large number of texts that can boost the managerial efficiency of this health facility when they are adapted, updated, or even reformed and rigorously applied. In addition to this approach, CHUY would benefit from using competent human resources, capable of leading its destiny and promoting the management of the hospital and university center.

5.3 The application of health legislation at the UHC

Except in cases of emergency, laws and regulations come into force as soon as they are promulgated or published. According to Article 2 of the Civil Code applicable in Cameroon, "the law is only for the future; it has no retroactive effect".) Laws and regulations, when they are not aimed at a particular object or person, have a general, abstract and even impartial scope. They apply to all individuals, which is why it is said that "no one is above the law". In general, the legislation is applied to UHC in a controversial manner. According to our sources, there are two main reasons for this controversial application of the legislation. The first reason is the incompetence of the human resources and the second is the bad faith of the latter. This means that the texts do not apply or at least are not applied properly at the CHUY. For our informants, the texts are more than ever poorly applied. In this regard, one respondent admitted that "if the CHUY is doing badly, it is because everyone is doing what they want. The legislation is more than ever poorly applied. In the same vein, other surveys found this application to be partial. There are many reasons for this poor application of health legislation at the UHC. Some informants mention ignorance of the legislation, which reflects the incompetence of CHUY's human resources. This is what one interviewee told us: "the poor application of health legislation is explained by the ignorance of the texts themselves, which reflects the incompetence of our leaders. However, on the first cover of the Cameroonian Penal Code it is written: "no one is supposed to ignore the law", even if we must recognize that there are more than 2000 laws and regulations.Owona (2013), already stated that many leaders make bad decisions because they do not have a good knowledge of the texts available in Cameroon. For the jurist, this was a good way to make people aware of the texts, because this simple knowledge can encourage compliance with the norm. This is all the more comfortable since Pasqua (2010) used this saying in these terms: "The old adage is still true: Fear of the police is the beginning of wisdom, but it is still necessary to see the police.[28]. Ondoa (2013) therefore proposed to resurrect the texts of Cameroon from 1815 to 2012[2929]. For the eminent law professor, texts are of notorious importance in a society. Borrowing the legal positivism of Kelsen, these texts must be protected, codified, standardized so that not only no one is unaware of them, but also so that we can make good use of them and especially that we can correct certain managerial practices, if necessary.Still on the subject of the reasons for the poor application of the legislation at the CHUY, other informants mentioned bad faith. For them, the texts are not normally applied not only because of simple ignorance, but also because the managers have no interest in applying them and sometimes because their interests are threatened. "It is above all bad faith that justifies this poor application of the texts," maintains an informant. From an observation retained in our grid, it emerges that the texts taken at the CHU Y do not respect the hierarchy of legal norms developed by Kelsen. Thus, a text adopted by the board of directors of this establishment is simply and purely rejected without further ado by the management of the CHUY. Such a way of doing things leads us to wonder whether an inferior norm could influence or prevail over a superior norm that conforms.Every behavior has consequences. These consequences can be negative or positive. At UHC, the poor application of health legislation seems to have a strong influence on the achievement of results. Indeed, this attitude constitutes an obstacle to the achievement of results. In our study, the majority of informants agree that results cannot be achieved at the CHUY in such a climate. Thus, our respondent number 4 is clear on this point: "the legislation as it is applied cannot allow CHUY to achieve results". According to the contingency school, the effectiveness o f an organization depends on activities such as: Planning, Organization, Personnel, Management, Coordination, Reporting and Budget. On the other hand, poor implementation of health legislation can throw one of these 7 activities off balance and prevent the achievement of results or better.However, the CHUY staff who made up our sample thought it would be better to restructure, reorient, reorganize, define a better legal framework for the health sector in general and the hospital sub-sector in particular, and above all to use competent human resources with integrity: "First of all, the hospital sub-sector must be restructured and reoriented, and then the legal system adapted to this sector must be harmonized to ensure that it is applied by people of integrity. This is the wish of one respondent. However, it should be noted that such an initiative is the responsibility of either the executive or the legislative branch, which is concurrently responsible for initiating laws[30]. It therefore requires the support or intervention of the State, as a regulatory body, for a better framing, or even a better organization of first category hospitals, and it is also necessary that the texts be applied. For it is only by applying the legislation that peace and serenity can reign in CHUY.

5.4 The effects of health legislation on the management of the University Hospital

To determine the effects of the health legislation on the management of CHUY, it was necessary to determine the type of management applicable in this health facility, its characteristics and to analyze the repercussions of the legislation, as it is applied, on the management of CHUY.Regarding the type of management applicable to UHC, let us first recall that there are several types of management. Secondly, it should be noted that there is no ideal type of management. The use of a particular type of management may depend on the circumstances, the socio-economic situation, the nature and size of the organization, the purpose and mission of the leader and even the personality of the leader. This last consideration, without taking into account all the others, seems to determine and characterize the management style of UHC in recent years. In fact, in our study, which focused on the impact of health legislation on the management of the CHUY, it emerged from the interviews with the staff in our sample that the management of this health establishment is directive in style. The directive management style is based on an organization established beforehand and imposed on the staff. Decision-making is the responsibility of the manager, who positions himself as a superior, expert and entitled to demand an immediate and effective response from his team. Throughout our various interviews with staff, some did not hesitate to clearly describe the management style of their hospital: "the management style is directive at the CHUY. The general management makes all the decisions. However, the CHUY is vast and this style is not appropriate", said respondent 1. For them, the directive style of management is not fruitful in a hospital as vast as the IUCY. This position is also shared by a large number of informants. UHC is a public hospital classified as an EPA. Its size and the large number of human resources it employs require a decentralized organization, a participatory management through which the leader associates and involves the personnel in the decision making process in a logic of delegation of power and ensures coordination. Mintzberg's theory of modeling relationships within an organization supports this view when it identifies 7 types of structures and 5 coordination mechanisms necessary for the coherence of actions carried out in an organization.Still in an effort to determine the management style of the CHUY, other informants stated strongly that it is authoritarian, dictatorial and even unclear for some. "The authoritarian style characterizes the management of the CHUY," one informant told us. According to another respondent. "It's a vague management", or even very unpleasant: "At the CHUY, it's a dictatorship" declared a distressed informant. However, all of these adjectives were in fact referring to the directive style. What is the characteristic of this management style at the CHUY?With regard to the characteristics of the management style, the data from our surveys show that the management of CHUY is chaotic, catastrophic, characterized by disorder, vagueness, and the cult of failure. These are the words used by our informants to characterize the managerial style of CHUY. Thus, one respondent did not hesitate to specify that "It is bad management, chaotic management similar to the management of the neighborhood grocery store. One informant simply repeated the terms used by Ateba Eyene: "It is a management of opacity". rereading the latter, we understand that the management of the CHUY is obscure and does not obey any existing standard. Such management cannot be profitable in an establishment such as the one in which the which served as a framework for our study.It is then necessary for the leaders of the CHUY to make an effective choice of the management style and to adapt it to the social, economic environment and even to each situation that would arise.The repercussions of health legislation on the management of the CHUY seem a little more frightening. Indeed, when legislation is poorly applied, its effects are very negative in the management of a hospital structure such as CHUY. This is all the more true since, in our survey, one informant took care to summarize these effects in these terms: "it is the poor functioning of the hospital, poor patient care, the absence of better supervision of students and better continuous training of staff". It should therefore be said that the legislation as it is applied at CHUY has resulted in the poor functioning of this health facility. Some disappointed informants even feel that it is not only the poor functioning, but above all the chaos of their hospital establishment. Finally, health legislation in general is intended to improve or even increase the performance of a given sector of activity. For this reason, it may convey norms aimed at organizing services or authorizing or prohibiting behavior. It is often said that where there are several individuals, rules must be established to govern their relationship, authorizing or prohibiting them from doing a particular act. At UHC, the controversial application of legislation can only produce controversial effects. It will not be consistent for such an attitude to produce positive effects. To confine this point of view, our informants recognize the purpose of health legislation to organize, regulate and allow the development of an activity or a sector, but the legislation applicable to CHUY can in no way have a positive impact on the management of this health and university training. The vast majority of the surveys unanimously share this position. One of them expressed it clearly in these terms: "Generally, the purpose of legislation is to organize and regulate a sector of activity. In this case, it has a positive impact on the management of the structure. However, its application at the CHUY produces negative effects in this hospital establishment".

CONCLUSION

Research on the impact of health legislation in the management of the CHUY is a major problem in the promotion of health and the care of patients in health facilities in Cameroon. For a very long time, health facilities in Cameroon have applied the technical watches left by the colon. Nowadays, the evolution of managerial techniques and the need for a better performance of health structures require a consideration of the health standards in force in our country.At CHUY, the staff seems to complain a lot about the management practiced by the leaders of this hospital and university institution. This led us to ask the question: "What is the impact of health legislation on the management of CHUY? The objective of this study was to analyze the impact of health legislation in the management of the said Center. The results of the survey showed that there is a multitude of legal texts applicable to health. These norms are intended to propel the managerial efficiency of the CHUY, provided that they are used properly. However, the application of legal norms is controversial at UHC Y. This misapplication of the legislation is justified by the incompetence of the human resources of CHUY and the bad faith of the management. This compromises the effectiveness, efficiency and achievement of expected results. It is therefore necessary to reorganize and improve the management of hospitals in Cameroon. This reorganization must emanate from the public authorities and consist in the reorganization of the Cameroonian health and hospital system. For the time being, the personnel must be competent and capable of leading or ensuring the respect and application of the existing health norms, necessary for the regulation of relations between men. In addition to resource allocation, the planning of activities not identified in our study, the hospital must function according to a certain cohesion between the caregivers of the same department, between the personnel of different departments, and then between the caregivers, patients and their families insofar as "most of the activity is governed by negotiations between the administrative structure and the care activity, between professional categories, within a professional category, between the professional world and the lay world, between t h e   hospital world and the outside world" (Carricâburu el Ménôret, 2004: 31). Thus, the health of an organization is defined on the basis of the degree of integration of the system it represents, the legal organization set up and it is the type of cultural orientation of the leader, his or her ideological choices that influence the type of hospital-patient relationships and the performance of that structure (Kuty, 1994). At the end of this study, we are far from feeling total satisfaction, as we recognize that some aspects of our survey were overlooked and could be the subject of future investigations. However, despite the results of this study, it is necessary to develop other similar research projects in other first class hospitals to deepen and complete these results and to have a legal framework capable of building a Cameroonian hospital paradise. This is why we insist on the project of a refoundation, an imperative reform of the Cameroonian health system and the hospital system for a better management of health conditions in Cameroon.

Table 25: Summary of suggestions

Concerned	Observations	Suggestions
Public authorities	Low autonomy of CHUY as an EPA	Reorganization of the decentralization of services in place of the deconcentration
	Lack of a general legal framework for first class hospitals	Standardization of legal texts in the health field, giving priority to a general orientation of hospital management and to the respect for the patient's rights
	Lack of hospital management tools	Definition of management tools based on RBM, GPEC and planning strategic
	Irrational use of available resources	Provide human, material and financial resources and ensure that they are managed as rationally as possibleci
	Low social security	The establishment of a real social security system for better care
		of health conditions in Cameroon
The administration of the CHUY	Weak adaptation of the CHUY in its legal hospital environment	Transmutation of the CHUY-EPA into a CHUY- EPPT with a special dispensation from the general status of EPAs, then reinforcement of the power of supervision over EPAs
	Weakness of the institutional framework	Updating of the procedure manual by clearly indicating the roles of each agent, in this case the Financial Controller, in fund disbursement operations
	The difficulty of achieving results	outcome planning and accountability of each agent through well-defined objectives

	Heavy interpersonal communication	Promote open collaboration and interpersonal communication and emphasize cultural and sports activities
	Use of available resources	Promote, internally, a more responsible management of resources and use of skills to achieve expected results
	High concentration of decisions	Decentralization and involvement of agents in the management of CHUY
	Inequalities	Promoting ethics, equity, justice and equality, see even ethics at UHC

Table 26: Survey Profile (ENQ.)

	Gender	Level of instruction	Function	Nature of commitment	seniority	Region of origin	Ethnicity
	M.	May sorting	Use of office	Contractual	14 years old	Center	Eton
	F	License	Head of department	Public servant	16 years old	East	Kako
	F	Doctoral student	Head of department	Contractual	14 years old	Coastal	Bonkeng
	M	Bac+TMS	Major	Contractual	32 years old	South	Fong
	M	License	Administrative framework	Contractual	27 years old	Center	Eton
	M	Bac+3	Nurse	Contractual	08 years old	Southwest	Bayangui
	F	Biological physician	Academic Physician	Public servant	05 years old	West	Bamiléké
	M	License	Administrative framework	Contractual	03 years old	South	Boulou
	M	Probatory	Accountant	Contractual	32 years old	Center	Ewondo
	M	Associate	Head of division	Public servant	26 years old	West	Bamoun
	F	Bac+3	Nurse	Public servant	12 years old	Center	Bassa
	M	CEP	Watchman	Contractual	08 years old	North	Mound Ang

Maintenance Guide

Hello !

I am ONANA Charles, student in Master II Hospital and Health Management at the School of Health Sciences of the Catholic University of Central Africa. As part of our training, we are required to submit a thesis for our Master's degree in Hospital and Health Management. Indeed, our theme is "The impact of health legislation on the management of the Yaoundé University Hospital". We kindly ask you to answer this interview guide in all sincerity. In this regard, we assure you that the information collected during this study will be used for purely scientific purposes in accordance with the provisions of Article 5 of Law No. 08/2009 on statistics. The information related to your identification (name(s), first name(s), phone number) is optional and confidential. So you won't have to worry about anything professionally. Would you like to participate? Thank you.

1- Respondent profiles

a) Gender;

b) Education Level;

c) Function;

d) Nature of the commitment;

e) Seniority;

f) Region of origin;

g) Ethnicity.

2. State of the art of health legislation at the CHUY

a) What do you think of the health legislation in Cameroon?

b) What can be said about the timeliness, adaptability and volume of the texts?

c) What is the capacity of health legislation to boost the managerial efficiency of CHUY?
d) What can be done to ensure that health legislation allows for the development of CHUY?

3. Application of health legislation at the UHC

a) What is your assessment of the application of health legislation at the UHC?

b) What can you say about the achievement of results with regard to the application of health legislation at UHC?
c) What needs to be done to improve health enforcement practices at UHC?

4. Effects of the health legislation on the management of the University Hospital

^{a)} What is the management style applicable to CHUY? What are the characteristics of this management style applied at CHUY? What are the implications of the health legislation) on UHC management? What is the impact of health legislation on the management of the UHC?

Thank you.

BIBLIOGRAPHIC REFERENCES

⬥ Ateba Eyene, C. (2010). The Management of Opacity and the Dramas of Cameroonian Society. Yaoundé: Edition Saint Paul.

⬥ Benoit, C. (2015). Manager un établissement de santé. Paris: Dalloz, 2nd edition,⬥ Braconnier, S. (2007). Droit des Services publics, 2ᵉ edition. Paris: PUF.

⬥ Carricaburu, D. & Ménoret, M. (2004). Sociology of health. Institutions. professions and diseases. Annan Colin, Coll. U Sociologie

⬥ Couture, C. and Lajeunesse, M. (1991). Archival Legislation and National Archival Policies: A Comparative Impact Study. Montreal, EBSÏ, (Research Report)

⬥ Crener, M. & Monteil, B. (1979). Principles of Management. Quebec: Presscs universitaires, Diffusion Vuibert

⬥ Dépelteau. F. (2000). La démarche d'une recherche en sciences humaines, Brussels: Presse de l'Université de Laval, De Boeck Université.

⬥ Drucker, P. (1984), Les entrepreneurs. Paris: Edition JC Lattes. Coll. L'Expansion Hachette December 1985.

⬥ Durkheim. E. (1960). On the Division of Social Work. Paris : PUF.

⬥ Fortin, M.F. (1996). Le processus de la recherche : de la conception à la réalisation.Ville Mont-Royal : Décaire Editeur.

⬥ Guillien, R. and Vincent, J. (1987). Lexique des termes juridiques. Paris: Dalloz.

⬥ Hart, J. & Sylvie (2002). Management hospitalier : Stratégies nouvelles des cadres. Paris : Edition LAMARRE, Collection Fondation Cadre Santé,

⬥ Hersey, P. & Blanchard, K.H. (1988). Management of organizational Behavior: Utilizing Human Resource. 5th ed. Englewood Cliffs, N J.: Prentice-Hall.

⬥ Holcman, R. (2015). Hospital management: a handbook of hospital governance and law. Paris: Dunod, Collection Guide d'action sociale,

⬥ Kelsen, H. (1992). What is the pure theory of law? In Droit et société, n°22. "Transformations of the State and legal changes: the example of Latin America".pp.   551-568.Retrieved on 16 October 2015 à at http://www.persee.fr/doc/dreso0769-3362 1992 number 22 1 1187

⬥ Kuty, O. (1994). Innovating in the hospital. Sociological analysis of a renal dialysis unit. Paris : l'harmattan.

⬥ Lexicon Of Legal Terms, 2013 Edition;

⬥ Manga Zambo, E. (2006). "The transformations of hospital management in their modern legal and administrative expressions in Cameroon". CAFRAD;

⬥ Mballa Owona, R. (2011). The notion of unilateral administrative act in Cameroon. Contribution to the theory of administrative decision. Saarbrücken: ÉditionsUniversitaires Européen nés.

⬥ Millard, E. (2006). General theory of law. Paris: Dalloz, Connaissance du droit.

⬥ Nkoum, B.A. (2005). Initiation à la recherche: une nécessité professionnelle. Yaoundé: UCAC Press.

⬥ Nobre, T. & Lambert P. (2012). Le management de pôles à l'hôpital Regards croisés, enjeux et défis. Paris : Denod.

🖶 Nobre, T. (2001). "Hospital management: from external control to steering, contribution and adaptability of the balanced scorecard". Comptabilité - Contrôle - Audit. Volume 7, p. 125-146.

🖶 Fayol, H. (1916). Industrial and general administration. Dunod, reed. 1962

🖶 NYEMB, G. (2012). Health Law, Ethics and Human Rights. Yaoundé: PUA.

🖶 Onana, C. (2015). "The legal responsibility of the hospital in Cameroon". InNkoum & Socpa, Cameroon's hospital at t h e time of managerial innovation.Yaoundé: UCAC Press. P.71-82

🖶 Ondoa, M. (2013), Texts and documents from Cameroon (1815 - 2012). Yaoundé : Editions le Kilimandjaro.

🖶 Roemer, R. (1998). "Health legislation: an instrument of public health and health policy. RILS, 49, 1: 85-97. Special issue on health legislation at the dawn of the 21st century, Geneva, WHO, XVII-289.

🖶 Sev S. Fluss (1998). "WHO's role in health legislation:historical overview". RILS, 49, 1: 85-97. Special Issue: Health Legislation in the 21st Century, Geneva, WHO, XVII.

🖶 Simo Kouam, F. A. (2015). " l a gouvernance hospitalière: condition d'efficacitémanagériale au Cameroun ". In Nkoum & Socpa. Cameroon's hospital at the time of managerial innovation^ Yaoundé : Presses de l'UCAC. P. 105-121

🖶 Vander Marren (2000). Dictionary of terms and concepts. Paris : Dalloz

🖶 Barnard, CI. (1938). The Functions of the Executive. Harvard University Press, ambridge, Mass. and London, 27th ed. 1976.

🖶 Daval, R. " Théorie des organisations ", Encyclopcedia Univer salis [en ligne], consulted on Thursday, 05 November 2015.URL: http://www.universalis.fr/encyclopedie/theorie-des-organisations

❖ **Legal texts**

🖶 The WHO Constitution (2006). in Basic Documents, Supplement to the Forty-fifth Edition, October 2006;

🖶 The law n° 74/18 of December 5, 1974 relating to the control of the authorizing officers and managers of public credits and companies;

🖶 The law n° 88/022 of December 16, 1988 modifying the law n° 84010 of December 5, 1984 fixing the organization of the order of the medical-health professions: nurse, midwife and medical-health technician;

🖶 Law No. 96/03 of January 4, 1996 on the Framework Law on Health;

🖶 The law n° 99/001 of April 7, 1999 relating to the exercise and the organization of the profession of optician;

🖶 Law N°2003/2006 of December 22, 2003 governing blood transfusion in Cameroon;

🖶 The decree N° 92 - 226 - PM of July 22, 1992 fixing the modalities of the control of the private medical formations;

🖶 Decree N° 94/303/PM of June 14, 1994 fixing the modalities of the quotas on the expensive transfers to certain medical and paramedical personnel practicing in the public medical formations;

- Decree No. 68/DF/419 of October 15, 1968 to determine the structural organization and the organic functioning of the hospital and health facilities in Cameroon,
- The decree N°2011/0004 of January 13, 2011 fixing the modalities of exercise of certain competences transferred by the State to the communes in terms of construction, equipment and management of the District Medical Centers;
- The decree, N°92-252-PM of July 6, 1992 fixing the conditions and the modalities of creation and opening of certain Private Health Trainings,
- Decrees n° 78/241 of June 24, 1978 and n° 91/065 of January 23, 1991 respectively on the creation and organization of a University Hospital Center (CHU).

- Laws n° 34 and 36 of August 10, 1990 respectively relating to the practice and organization of the medical profession in Cameroon and to the practice of profession of dental surgeon;

- WHO, (2005), International Health Regulations, Second Edition

TABLE OF CONTENTS

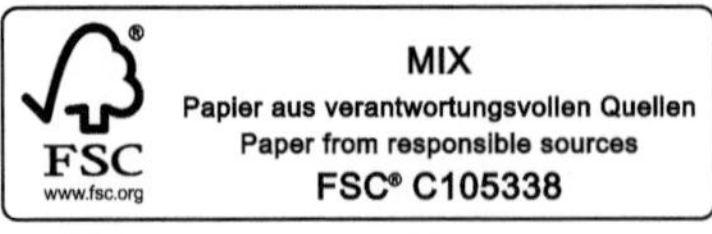

Printed by Books on Demand GmbH, Norderstedt / Germany